ANTI-INFLAMMATORY COOKBOOK 2022

DELICIOUS AND QUICK RECIPES
TO RESTORE YOUR HEALTH
FOR BEGINNERS

JESSICA STEIN

Table of Contents

Spiced Broccoli, Cauliflower, And Tofu With Red Onion 16
Ingredients: 16
Directions: 17
Beans And Salmon Pan Servings: 4 18
Ingredients: 18
Directions: 19
Carrot Soup Servings: 4 20
Ingredients: 20
Directions: 21
Healthy Pasta Salad Servings: 6 22
Ingredients: 22
Directions: 22
Chickpea Curry Servings: 4 To 6 24
Ingredients: 24
Directions: 25
Ground Meat Stroganoff Ingredients: 26
Directions: 26
Saucy Short Ribs Servings: 4 28
Ingredients: 28
Directions: 29
Chicken And Gluten-free Noodle Soup Servings: 4 30
Ingredients: 30
Lentil Curry Servings: 4 32
Ingredients: 32

- Directions: 33
- Chicken And Snap Pea Stir-fry Servings: 4 34
- Ingredients: 34
- Directions: 35
- Juicy Broccolini With Anchovy Almonds Servings: 6 36
- Ingredients: 36
- Directions: 36
- Shiitake And Spinach Pattie Servings: 8 38
- Ingredients: 38
- Directions: 39
- Broccoli Cauliflower Salad Servings: 6 40
- Ingredients: 40
- Directions: 41
- Chicken Salad With Chinese Touch Servings: 3 42
- Ingredients: 42
- Directions: 43
- Amaranth And Quinoa Stuffed Peppers Servings: 4 44
- Ingredients: 44
- Crispy Cheese-crusted Fish Fillet Servings: 4 46
- Ingredients: 46
- Directions: 46
- Protein Power Beans And Green Stuffed Shells 48
- Ingredients: 48
- Asian Noodle Salad Ingredients: 51
- Directions: 51
- Salmon And Green Beans Servings: 4 53
- Ingredients: 53

Directions: 53

Cheesy Stuffed Chicken Ingredients: 55

Directions: 56

Arugula With Gorgonzola Dressing Servings: 4 57

Ingredients: 57

Directions: 57

Cabbage Soup Servings: 6 59

Ingredients: 59

Cauliflower Rice Servings: 4 60

Ingredients: 60

Directions: 60

Feta Frittata & Spinach Servings: 4 61

Ingredients: 61

Directions: 61

Fiery Chicken Pot Stickers Ingredients: 63

Directions: 64

Garlic Shrimps With Gritted Cauliflower Servings: 2 65

Ingredients: 65

Directions: 66

Broccoli Tuna Servings: 1 67

Ingredients: 67

Directions: 67

Butternut Squash Soup With Shrimp Servings: 4 68

Ingredients: 68

Directions: 69

Tasty Turkey Baked Balls Servings: 6 70

Ingredients: 70

- Directions: 70
- Clear Clam Chowder Servings: 4 72
- Ingredients: 72
- Directions: 73
- Rice And Chicken Pot Servings: 4 74
- Ingredients: 74
- Directions: 75
- Sautéed Shrimp Jambalaya Jumble Servings: 4 77
- Ingredients: 77
- Chicken Chili Servings: 6 79
- Ingredients: 79
- Directions: 80
- Garlic And Lentil Soup Servings: 4 81
- Ingredients: 81
- Zesty Zucchini & Chicken In Classic Santa Fe Stir-fry 83
- Ingredients: 83
- Directions: 84
- Tilapia Tacos With Awesome Ginger-sesame Slaw 85
- Ingredients: 85
- Directions: 85
- Curry Lentil Stew Servings: 4 87
- Ingredients: 87
- Directions: 87
- Kale Caesar Salad With Grilled Chicken Wrap Servings: 2 89
- Ingredients: 89
- Directions: 90
- Spinach Bean Salad Servings: 1 91

Ingredients:	91
Directions:	91
Crusted Salmon With Walnuts & Rosemary Servings: 6	92
Ingredients:	92
Directions:	93
Baked Sweet Potato With Red Tahini Sauce Servings: 4	94
Ingredients:	94
Directions:	95
Italian Summer Squash Soup Servings: 4	96
Ingredients:	96
Directions:	97
Saffron And Salmon Soup Servings: 4	98
Ingredients:	98
Thai Flavored Hot And Sour Shrimp And Mushroom Soup	100
Ingredients:	100
Directions:	101
Orzo With Sundried Tomatoes Ingredients:	102
Directions:	102
Mushroom And Beet Soup Servings: 4	104
Ingredients:	104
Directions:	104
Chicken Parmesan Meatballs Ingredients:	106
Directions:	106
Meatballs Alla Parmigiana Ingredients:	108
Directions:	109
Sheet Pan Turkey Breast With Golden Vegetables	110
Ingredients:	110

Directions: 110

Coconut Green Curry With Boil Rice Servings: 8 112

Ingredients: 112

Directions: 112

Sweet Potato & Chicken Soup With Lentil Servings: 6 114

Ingredients: 114

Directions: 115

Creamy Pork And Tomatoes Servings: 4 116

Ingredients: 116

Directions: 116

Lemon Tenderloin Servings: 2 118

Ingredients: 118

Chicken With Broccoli Servings: 4 120

Ingredients: 120

Directions: 120

Crispy Chicken Tenderloin Servings: 4 121

Ingredients: 121

Directions: 121

Pork With Mushrooms And Cucumbers Servings: 4 122

Ingredients: 122

Directions: 122

Chicken Chopstick Servings: 4 124

Ingredients: 124

Directions: 124

Balsamic Roast Chicken Servings: 4 126

Ingredients: 126

Directions: 126

Steak & Mushrooms Servings: 4 128

Ingredients: 128

Directions: 128

Beef Tips Servings: 4 129

Ingredients: 129

Directions: 129

Peach Chicken Treat Servings: 4-5 131

Ingredients: 131

Directions: 131

Ground Pork Pan Servings: 4 133

Ingredients: 133

Directions: 134

Parsley Pork And Artichokes Servings: 4 135

Ingredients: 135

Directions: 136

Pork With Thyme Sweet Potatoes Servings: 4 137

Ingredients: 137

Directions: 138

Curry Pork Mix Servings: 4 139

Ingredients: 139

Directions: 139

Stir-fried Chicken And Broccoli Servings: 4 141

Ingredients: 141

Directions: 141

Chicken And Broccoli Servings: 4 143

Ingredients: 143

Directions: 144

Mediterranean Chicken Bake With Vegetables Servings: 4 145

Ingredients: 145

Directions: 145

Hidden Valley Chicken Drummies Servings: 6 - 8 147

Ingredients: 147

Directions: 147

Balsamic Chicken And Beans Servings: 4 149

Ingredients: 149

Directions: 149

Italian Pork Servings: 6 151

Ingredients: 151

Directions: 152

Chicken And Brussels Sprouts Servings: 4 153

Ingredients: 153

Directions: 153

Chicken Divan Ingredients: 154

Directions: 154

Parmesan Chicken Servings: 4 155

Ingredients: 155

Directions: 155

Sumptuous Indian Chicken Curry Servings: 6 157

Ingredients: 157

Directions: 158

Pork With Balsamic Onion Sauce Servings: 4 160

Ingredients: 160

Directions: 160

Ingredients: 161

Directions: 162

Pork With Pears And Ginger Servings: 4 163

Ingredients: 163

Directions: 163

Butter Chicken Servings: 6 165

Ingredients: 165

Directions: 165

Hot Chicken Wings Servings: 4 - 5 166

Ingredients: 166

Directions: 166

Chicken, Pasta And Snow Peas Servings: 1 - 2 167

Ingredients: 167

Directions: 167

Ingredients: 168

Directions: 169

Apricot Chicken Wings Servings: 3 - 4 170

Ingredients: 170

Directions: 170

Chicken Thighs Servings: 4 172

Ingredients: 172

Directions: 172

Crispy Chicken Tenders Servings: 4 173

Ingredients: 173

Directions: 173

Champion Chicken Pockets Servings: 4 175

Ingredients: 175

Directions: 175

Stovetop Barbecued Chicken Bites Servings: 4 176
Ingredients: 176
Directions: 177
Chicken And Radish Mix Servings: 4 178
Ingredients: 178
Directions: 178
Chicken Katsu Servings: 4 179
Ingredients: 179
Directions: 180
Chicken And Sweet Potato Stew Servings: 4 181
Ingredients: 181
Directions: 181
Rosemary Beef Ribs Servings: 4 183
Ingredients: 183
Directions: 183
Chicken, Bell Pepper & Spinach Frittata Servings: 8 185
Ingredients: 185
Directions: 185
Roast Chicken Dal Servings: 4 187
Ingredients: 187
Directions: 187
Chicken Taquitos Servings: 6 189
Ingredients: 189
Directions: 189
Oregano Pork Servings: 4 191
Ingredients: 191
Directions: 192

Chicken And Avocado Bake Servings: 4 193
Ingredients: 193
Directions: 193
Five-spice Roasted Duck Breasts Servings: 4 195
Ingredients: 195
Directions: 195
Pork Chops With Tomato Salsa Servings: 4 197
Ingredients: 197
Directions: 198
Tuscan Chicken With Tomatoes, Olives, And Zucchini 199
Ingredients: 199
Directions: 200
Pork Salad Servings: 4 201
Ingredients: 201
Directions: 202
Lime Pork And Green Beans Servings: 4 203
Ingredients: 203
Directions: 204
Chicken Breast Servings: 4 205
Ingredients: 205
Directions: 205
Pork With Chili Zucchinis And Tomatoes Servings: 4 206
Ingredients: 206
Directions: 207
Pork With Olives Servings: 4 208
Ingredients: 208
Directions: 208

Dill And Salmon Pâté 210

Ingredients: 210

Directions: 210

Chai Spice Baked Apples Servings: 5 211

Ingredients: 211

Directions: 211

Peach Crisp Servings: 6 213

Ingredients: 213

Directions: 213

Peach Dip Servings: 2 215

Ingredients: 215

Directions: 215

Carrot And Pumpkin Seed Crackers Servings: 40 Crackers 216

Ingredients: 216

Directions: 216

Avocado Fries Servings: 8 218

Ingredients: 218

Directions: 219

Spiced Broccoli, Cauliflower, And Tofu With Red Onion

Servings: 2

Cooking Time: 25 Minutes

Ingredients:

2 cups broccoli florets

2 cups cauliflower florets

1 medium red onion, diced

3 tablespoons extra-virgin olive oil

1 teaspoon salt

¼ teaspoon freshly ground black pepper

1-pound firm tofu, cut into 1-inch dice

1 garlic clove, minced

1 (¼-inch) piece fresh ginger, minced

Directions:

1. Preheat the oven to 400°F.

2. Combine the broccoli, cauliflower, onion, oil, salt, and pepper on a large rimmed baking sheet, and mix well.

3. Roast until the vegetables have softened, 10 to 15 minutes.

4. Add the tofu, garlic, and ginger. Roast within 10 minutes.

5. Gently mix the ingredients on the baking sheet to combine the tofu with the vegetables and serve.

<u>Nutrition Info:</u> Calories 210 Total Fat: 15g Total Carbohydrates: 11g Sugar: 4g Fiber: 4g Protein: 12g Sodium: 626mg

Beans And Salmon Pan *Servings: 4*

Cooking Time: 25 Minutes

Ingredients:

1 cup canned black beans, drained and rinsed 4 garlic cloves, minced

1 yellow onion, chopped

2 tablespoons olive oil

4 salmon fillets, boneless

½ teaspoon coriander, ground

1 teaspoon turmeric powder

2 tomatoes, cubed

½ cup chicken stock

A pinch of salt and black pepper

½ teaspoon cumin seeds

1 tablespoon chives, chopped

Directions:

1. Heat up a pan with the oil over medium heat, add the onion and the garlic and sauté for 5 minutes.

2. Add the fish and sear it for 2 minutes on each side.

3. Add the beans and the other ingredients, toss gently and cook for 10 minutes more.

4. Divide the mix between plates and serve right away for lunch.

Nutrition Info: calories 219, fat 8, fiber 8, carbs 12, protein 8

Carrot Soup _Servings: 4_

Cooking Time: 40 Minutes

Ingredients:

1 cup Butternut Squash, chopped

1 tbsp. Olive Oil

1 tbsp. Turmeric Powder

14 ½ oz. Coconut Milk, light

3 cups Carrot, chopped

1 Leek, rinsed & sliced

1 tbsp. Ginger, grated

3 cups Vegetable Broth

1 cup Fennel, chopped

Salt & Pepper, to taste

2 cloves of Garlic, minced

Directions:

1. Start by heating a Dutch oven over medium-high heat.

2. To this, spoon in the oil and then stir in fennel, squash, carrots, and leek. Mix well.

3. Now, sauté it for 4 to 5 minutes or until softened.

4. Next, add turmeric, ginger, pepper, and garlic to it. Cook for another 1 to 2 minutes.

5. Then, pour the broth and coconut milk to it. Combine well.

6. After that, bring the mixture to a boil and cover the Dutch oven.

7. Allow it to simmer for 20 minutes.

8. Once cooked, transfer the mixture to a high-speed blender and blend for 1 to 2 minutes or until you get a creamy smooth soup.

9. Check for seasoning and spoon in more salt and pepper if needed.

Nutrition Info: Calories: 210.4KcalProteins: 2.11gCarbohydrates: 25.64gFat: 10.91g

Healthy Pasta Salad _Servings: 6_

Cooking Time: 10 Minutes

Ingredients:

1 package of gluten-free fusilli pasta

1 cup of grape tomatoes, sliced

1 handful of fresh cilantro, chopped

1 cup of olives, halved

1 cup of fresh basil, chopped

½ cup of olive oil

Sea salt to taste

Directions:

1. Whisk together the olive oil, chopped basil, cilantro, and sea salt. Set aside.

2. Cook the pasta according to package directions, strain, and rinse.

3. Combine the pasta with the tomatoes and olives.

4. Add the olive oil mixture, and toss until well combined.

Nutrition Info: Total Carbohydrates 66g Dietary Fiber: 5g Protein: 13g Total Fat: 23g Calories: 525

Chickpea Curry _Servings: 4 To 6_

Cooking Time: 25 Minutes

Ingredients:

2 × 15 oz. Chickpeas, washed, drained & cooked 2 tbsp. Olive Oil

1 tbsp. Turmeric Powder

½ of 1 Onion, diced

1 tsp. Cayenne, grounded

4 Garlic cloves, minced

2 tsp. Chili Powder

15 oz. Tomato Puree

Black Pepper, as needed

2 tbsp. Tomato Paste

1 tsp. Cayenne, grounded

½ tbsp. Maple Syrup

½ of 15 oz. can of Coconut Milk

2 tsp. Cumin, grounded

2 tsp. Smoked Paprika

Directions:

1. Heat a large skillet over medium-high heat. To this, spoon in the oil.

2. Once the oil becomes hot, stir in the onion and cook for 3 to 4 minutes or until softened.

3. Next, spoon in the tomato paste, maple syrup, all seasonings, tomato puree, and garlic into it. Mix well.

4. Then, add the cooked chickpeas to it along with coconut milk, black pepper, and salt.

5. Now, give everything a good stir and allow it to simmer for 8 to 10 minutes or until thickened.

6. Drizzle lime juice over it and garnish with cilantro, if desired.

Nutrition Info: Calories: 224KcalProteins: 15.2gCarbohydrates: 32.4gFat: 7.5g

Ground Meat Stroganoff_Ingredients:

1 lb lean ground meat

1 little onion diced

1 clove garlic minced

3/4 lb new mushrooms cut

3 tablespoons flour

2 cups meat stock

salt and pepper to taste

2 teaspoons Worcestershire sauce

3/4 cup sharp cream

2 tablespoons new parsley

Directions:

1. Dark colored ground hamburger, onion and garlic (making an effort not to split it up something over the top) in a dish until no pink remains. Channel fat.

2. Include cut mushrooms and cook 2-3 minutes. Mix in flour and cook 1 progressively minute.

3. Include stock, Worcestershire sauce, salt and pepper and heat to the point of boiling. Lessen warmth and stew on low 10 minutes.

Cook egg noodles as indicated by bundle headings.

4. Expel meat blend from the warmth, mix in sharp cream and parsley.

5. Serve over egg noodles.

Saucy Short Ribs *Servings: 4*

Cooking Time: 65 Minutes

Ingredients:

2 lbs. beef short ribs

1 ½ tsp olive oil

1 ½ tbsp soy sauce

1 tbsp Worcestershire sauce

1 tbsp stevia

1 ¼ cups onion chopped.

1 tsp garlic minced

1/2 cup red wine

⅓ cup ketchup, sugar-free

Salt and black pepper to taste

Directions:

1. Slice the ribs into 3 segments and rub them with black pepper and salt.

2. Add oil to the Instant Pot and hit Sauté.

3. Place the ribs in the oil and sear for 5 minutes per side.

4. Toss in onion and sauté for 4 minutes.

5. Stir in garlic and cook for 1 minute.

6. Whisk rest of the ingredients in a bowl and pour over the ribs.

7. Put on its pressure lid and cook for 55 minutes on Manual mode at High pressure.

8. Once done, release the pressure naturally then remove the lid.

9. Serve warm.

Nutrition Info: Calories 555, Carbs 12.8g, Protein 66.7g, Fat 22.3g, Fiber 0.9g

Chicken And Gluten-free Noodle Soup **Servings: 4**

Cooking Time: 25 Minutes

Ingredients:

¼ cup extra-virgin olive oil

3 celery stalks, cut into ¼-inch slices

2 medium carrots, cut into ¼-inch dice

1 small onion, cut into ¼-inch dice

1 fresh rosemary sprig

4 cups chicken broth

8 ounces gluten-free penne

1 teaspoon salt

¼ teaspoon freshly ground black pepper

2 cups diced rotisserie chicken

¼ cup finely chopped fresh flat-leaf parsley Directions:

1. Heat-up the oil over high heat in a large pot.

2. Put the celery, carrots, onion, and rosemary and sauté until softened, 5 to 7 minutes.

3. Add the broth, penne, salt, and pepper and boil.

4. Simmer and cook until the penne is tender, 8 to 10 minutes.

5. Remove and discard the rosemary sprig, and add the chicken and parsley.

6. Reduce the heat to low. Cook within 5 minutes, and serve.

Nutrition Info: Calories 485 Total Fat: 18g Total Carbohydrates: 47g Sugar: 4g Fiber: 7g Protein: 33g Sodium: 1423mg

Lentil Curry _Servings: 4_

Cooking Time: 40 Minutes

Ingredients:

2 tsp. Mustard Seeds

1 tsp. Turmeric, grounded

1 cup Lentils, soaked

2 tsp. Cumin Seeds

1 Tomato, large & chopped

1 Yellow Onion, sliced finely

4 cups Water

Sea Salt, as needed

2 Carrots, sliced into half-moons

3 handful of Spinach leaves, shredded

1 tsp. Ginger, minced

½ tsp. Chili Powder

2 tbsp. Coconut Oil

Directions:

1. First, place the mung beans and water in a deep saucepan over medium-high heat.

2. Now, bring the beans mixture to a boil and allow it to simmer.

3. Simmer within 20 to 30 minutes or until the mung beans are softened.

4. Then, heat the coconut oil in a large saucepan over medium heat and stir in the mustard seeds and cumin seeds.

5. If the mustard seeds pop, put the onions. Sauté the onions for 4 minutes or until they softened.

6. Spoon in the garlic and continue sautéing for another 1 minute. Once aromatic, spoon in the turmeric and chili powder to it.

7. Then, add the carrot and tomato—Cook for 6 minutes or until softened.

8. Finally, add the cooked lentils to it and give everything a good stir.

9. Stir in the spinach leaves and sauté until wilted. Remove from heat. Serve it warm and enjoy.

Nutrition Info: Calories 290Kcal Proteins: 14g Carbohydrates: 43g Fat: 8g

Chicken And Snap Pea Stir-fry Servings: 4

Cooking Time: 10 Minutes

Ingredients:

1 ¼ cups boneless skinless chicken breast, thinly sliced 3 tablespoons fresh cilantro, chopped

2 tablespoons vegetable oil

2 tablespoons of sesame seeds

1 bunch scallions, thinly sliced

2 teaspoons Sriracha

2 garlic cloves, minced

2 tablespoons rice vinegar

1 bell pepper, thinly sliced

3 tablespoons soy sauce

2½ cups snap peas

Salt, to taste

Freshly ground black pepper, to taste

Directions:

1. Heat-up the oil in a pan over medium heat. Add garlic and thinly sliced scallions. Cook for a minute and then add 2 ½ cups snap peas along with bell pepper. Cook until tender, just for about 3-4 minutes.

2. Add chicken and cook for about 4-5 minutes, or until thoroughly cooked.

3. Add in 2 teaspoons Sriracha, 2 tablespoons of sesame seeds, 3

tablespoons soy sauce, and 2 tablespoons rice vinegar. Toss everything until well-combined. Simmer within 2-3 minutes over low heat.

4. Add 3 tablespoons of chopped cilantro and stir well. Transfer, and sprinkle with extra sesame seeds and cilantro, if needed. Enjoy!

<u>Nutrition Info:</u> 228 calories 11 g fat 11 g total carbs 20 g protein

Juicy Broccolini With Anchovy Almonds

Servings: 6

Cooking Time: 10 Minutes

Ingredients:

2 bunches of broccolini, trimmed

1 tablespoon extra-virgin olive oil

1 long fresh red chili, deseeded, finely chopped 2 garlic cloves, thinly sliced

¼ cup natural almonds, coarsely chopped

2 teaspoons lemon rind, finely grated

A squeeze of lemon juice, fresh

4 anchovies in oil, chopped

Directions:

1. Warm the oil until hot in a large saucepan. Add the drained anchovies, garlic, chili, and lemon rind. Cook until aromatic, for 30 seconds, stirring frequently. Add the almond & continue to cook for a minute more, stirring frequently. Remove from the heat & add a squeeze of fresh lemon juice.

2. Then place the broccolini in a steamer basket set over a saucepan of simmering water. Cover & cook until crisp-tender, for 2

to 3 minutes. Drain well and then transfer to a large-sized serving plate. Top with the almond mixture. Enjoy.

Nutrition Info: kcal 350 Fat: 7 g Fiber: 3 g Protein: 6 g

Shiitake And Spinach Pattie *Servings: 8*

Cooking Time: 15 Minutes

Ingredients:

1 ½ cups shiitake mushrooms, minced

1 ½ cups spinach, chopped

3 garlic cloves, minced

2 onions, minced

4 tsp. olive oil

1 egg

1 ½ cups quinoa, cooked

1 ½ tsp. Italian seasoning

1/3 cup toasted sunflower seeds, ground

1/3 cup Pecorino cheese, grated

Directions:

1. Heat olive oil in a saucepan. Once hot, sauté shiitake mushrooms for 3 minutes or until lightly seared. Add in garlic and onion. Sauté for 2 minutes or until fragrant and translucent. Set aside.

2. In the same saucepan, heat the remaining olive oil. Add in spinach. Reduce heat, then simmer for 1 minute, drain and transfer to a strainer.

3. Chop spinach finely and add into the mushroom mixture. Add egg into the spinach mixture. Fold in cooked quinoa—season with Italian seasoning, then mix until well combined. Sprinkle sunflower seeds and cheese.

4. Divide the spinach mixture into patties—Cook patties within 5

minutes or until firm and golden brown. Serve with burger bread.

Nutrition Info: Calories 43 Carbs: 9g Fat: 0g Protein: 3g

Broccoli Cauliflower Salad <u>Servings: 6</u>

Cooking Time: 20 Minutes

Ingredients:

¼ tsp. Black Pepper, grounded

3 cups Cauliflower Florets

1 tbsp. Vinegar

1 tsp. Honey

8 cups Kale, chopped

3 cups Broccoli Florets

4 tbsp. Extra Virgin Olive Oil

½ tsp. Salt

1 ½ tsp. Dijon Mustard

1 tsp. Honey

½ cup Cherries, dried

1/3 cup Pecans, chopped

1 cup Manchego cheese, shaved

Directions:

1. Preheat the oven to 450 ° F and place a baking sheet in the middle rack.

2. After that, place cauliflower and broccoli florets in a large bowl.

3. To this, spoon in half of the salt, two tablespoons of the oil and pepper. Toss well.

4. Now, transfer the mixture to the preheated sheet and bake it for 12 minutes while flipping it once in between.

5. Once it becomes tender and golden in color, remove it from the oven and allow it to cool completely.

6. In the meantime, mix the remaining two tablespoons of oil, vinegar, honey, mustard, and salt in another bowl.

7. Brush this mixture over the kale leaves by messaging the leaves with your hands. Set it aside for 3 to 5 minutes.

8. Finally, stir in the roasted vegetables, cheese, cherries, and pecan to the broccoli-cauliflower salad.

<u>Nutrition Info:</u> Calories: 259KcalProteins: 8.4gCarbohydrates: 23.2gFat: 16.3g

Chicken Salad With Chinese Touch *Servings: 3*

Cooking Time: 25 Minutes

Ingredients:

1 Medium green onion (thinly sliced)

2 Boneless chicken breasts

2tbsp Soya sauce

¼ Teaspoon white pepper

1tbsp sesame oil

4 cups romaine lettuce (chopped)

1 cup cabbage (shredded)

¼ Cup small cubes carrots

¼ Cup thin sliced almonds

¼ Cup noodles (only for serving)

For Preparing Chinese Dressing:

1 Minced garlic clove

1 Teaspoon soy sauce

1tbsp sesame oil

2tbsp Rice vinegar

1tbsp Sugar

Directions:

1. Prepare Chinese dressing by whisking all ingredients in a bowl.

2. In a bowl, marinate chicken breasts with garlic, olive oil, soy sauce, and white pepper for 20 minutes.

3. Place baking dish in the preheated oven (at 225C).

4. Place chicken breasts in the baking dish and bake it almost for 20 minutes.

5. For assembling the salad, combine romaine lettuce, cabbage, carrots, and green onion.

6. For serving, place a chicken piece in a plate and salad on top of it. Pour some dressing over it alongside noodles.

Nutrition Info: Calories 130 Carbs: 10g Fat: 6g Protein: 10g

Amaranth And Quinoa Stuffed Peppers

Servings: 4

Cooking Time: 1 Hour & 10 Minutes

Ingredients:

2 tablespoons Amaranth

1 medium zucchini, trimmed, grated

2 vine-ripened tomatoes, diced

2/3 cup (approximately 135 g) quinoa

1 onion, medium-sized, chopped finely

2 crushed garlic cloves

1 teaspoon ground cumin

2 tablespoons lightly toasted sunflower seeds 75g ricotta cheese, fresh

2 tablespoons currants

4 capsicums, large, halved lengthwise & seeded 2 tablespoons flat-leaf parsley, roughly chopped Directions:

1. Line a baking tray, preferably large-sized with some baking paper (nonstick) and then preheat your oven to 350 F in advance. Fill a medium-

sized saucepan with an approximately a half-liter of water and then add the amaranth and quinoa; bring it to a boil over moderate heat. Once done, decrease the heat to low; cover & let simmer until grains turn al dente and water is absorbed, for 12 to 15

minutes. Remove from the heat & set aside.

2. In the meantime, lightly coat a large-sized frying pan with oil and heat it over medium heat. Once hot, add the onion with zucchini & cook until softened, for a couple of minutes, stirring frequently. Add the cumin and garlic; cook for a minute. Remove from the heat & set aside to cool.

3. Place the grains, onion mixture, sunflower seeds, currants, parsley, ricotta, and tomato in a mixing bowl, preferably large-sized; give the ingredients a good stir until combined well—season with pepper and salt to taste.

4. Fill the capsicums with prepared quinoa mixture & arrange them on the tray, covering the tray with aluminum foil—Bake for 17 to 20

minutes. Remove the foil & bake until the stuffing turns into golden & vegetables turn fork-tender, for 15 to 20 more minutes.

Nutrition Info: kcal 200 Fat: 8.5 g Fiber: 8 g Protein: 15 g

Crispy Cheese-crusted Fish Fillet _Servings: 4_

Cooking Time: 10 Minutes

Ingredients:

¼-cup whole-wheat breadcrumbs

¼-cup Parmesan cheese, grated

¼-tsp sea salt ¼-tsp ground pepper

1-Tbsp. olive oil 4-pcs tilapia fillets

Directions:

1. Preheat the oven to 375°F.

2. Stir in the breadcrumbs, Parmesan cheese, salt, pepper, and olive oil in a mixing bowl.

3. Mix well until blended thoroughly.

4. Coat the fillets with the mixture, and lay each on a lightly sprayed baking sheet.

5. Place the sheet in the oven.

6. Bake for 10 minutes until the fillets cook through and turn brownish.

Nutrition Info: Calories: 255Fat: 7gProtein: 15.9gCarbs: 34gFiber: 2.6g

Protein Power Beans And Green Stuffed Shells

Ingredients:

Genuine or ocean salt

Olive oil

12 oz. bundle kind sized shells (around 40) 1 lb. solidified cleaved spinach

2 to 3 cloves garlic, stripped and divided

15 to 16 oz. ricotta cheddar (ideally full fat/entire milk) 2 eggs

1 can white beans, (for example, cannellini), depleted and flushed

½ C green pesto, custom made or locally acquired Ground dark pepper

3 C (or more) marinara sauce

Ground parmesan or pecorino cheddar (discretionary) <u>Directions:</u>

1. Heat at any rate 5 quarts of water to the point of boiling in an enormous pot (or work in two littler clumps). Include a tablespoon of salt, a sprinkle of olive oil, and the shells. Bubble around 9 minutes (or until extremely still somewhat firm), blending sporadically to keep the shells isolated. Tenderly channel the shells in a colander, or scoop from the water with an opened spoon. Wash quickly with cool water. Line a rimmed heating sheet with cling wrap. At the point when the shells are sufficiently cool to deal with,

separate them by hand, dumping out extra water and putting opening up in a solitary layer on the sheet container. Spread with progressively plastic wrap once practically cool.

2. Bring a couple of quarts of water (or utilize remaining pasta water, on the off chance that you didn't dump it out) to a bubble in a similar pot. Include solidified spinach and cook three minutes on high, until delicate. Line the colander with soggy paper towels on the off chance that the openings are enormous, at that point channel the spinach. Set colander over a bowl to deplete more while you start the filling.

3. Add only the garlic to a nourishment processor and run until it's finely hacked and adhering to the sides. Scratch down the sides of the bowl, at that point include the ricotta, eggs, beans, pesto, 1½

teaspoons salt, and a few toils of pepper (a major squeeze). Press the spinach in your grasp to deplete well of outstanding water, at that point add to different fixings in the nourishment processor. Run until practically smooth, with a couple of little bits of spinach still noticeable. I lean toward not to taste subsequent to including the crude egg, yet on the off chance that you think that its fundamental taste a little and modify flavoring to taste.

4. Preheat the broiler to 350 (F) and shower or gently oil a 9 x 13"

skillet, in addition to another littler goulash dish (around 8 to 10 of the shells won't fit in the 9 x 13). To fill the shells, get each shell in turn, holding it open with thumb and pointer finger of your non-predominant hand.

Scoop 3 to 4 tablespoons loading up with your other hand and scratch into the shell. The greater part of them won't look great, which is alright! Spot filled shells near one another in the readied container. Spoon sauce over the shells, leaving bits of the green filling unmistakable. Spread container with thwart and prepare for 30 minutes. Increment warmth to 375 (F), sprinkle shells with some ground parmesan (if utilizing), and heat revealed for another 5

to 10 minutes until cheddar is dissolved and abundance dampness is diminished.

5. Cool 5 to 10 minutes, at that point serve alone or with a fresh plate of mixed greens as an afterthought!

Asian Noodle Salad Ingredients:

8 ounces in length slight entire wheat pasta noodles —, for example, spaghetti (use soba noodles to make gluten free) 24 ounces Mann's Broccoli Cole Slaw — 2 12-ounce sacks 4 ounces ground carrots

1/4 cup extra-virgin olive oil

1/4 cup rice vinegar

3 tablespoons nectar — utilize light agave nectar to make veggie lover

3 tablespoons smooth nutty spread

2 tablespoons low-sodium soy sauce — gluten free if necessary 1 tablespoon Sriracha pepper sauce — or garlic chile sauce, in addition to extra to taste

1 tablespoon minced new ginger

2 teaspoons minced garlic — around 4 cloves 3/4 cup broiled unsalted peanuts, — generally slashed 3/4 cup new cilantro — finely slashed

Directions:

1. Heat a huge pot of salted water to the point of boiling. Cook the noodles until still somewhat firm, as per bundle headings. Channel and flush quickly with cool water to evacuate the overabundance starch and stop the

cooking, at that point move to a huge serving bowl. Include the broccoli cole slaw and carrots.

2. While the pasta cooks, whisk together the olive oil, rice vinegar, nectar, nutty spread, soy sauce, Sriarcha, ginger, and garlic. Pour over the noodle blend and hurl to consolidate. Include the peanuts and cilantro and hurl again. Serve chilled or at room temperature with extra Sriracha sauce as wanted.

3. Formula Notes

4. Asian Noodle Salad can be served cold or at room temperature.

Store remains in the cooler in a water/air proof holder for as long as 3 days.

Salmon And Green Beans *Servings: 4*

Cooking Time: 26 Minutes

Ingredients:

2 tablespoons olive oil

1 yellow onion, chopped

4 salmon fillets, boneless

1 cup green beans, trimmed and halved

2 garlic cloves, minced

½ cup chicken stock

1 teaspoon chili powder

1 teaspoon sweet paprika

A pinch of salt and black pepper

1 tablespoon cilantro, chopped

Directions:

1. Heat up a pan with the oil over medium heat, add onion, stir and sauté for 2 minutes.

2. Add the fish and sear it for 2 minutes on each side.

3. Add the rest of the ingredients, toss gently and bake everything at 360 degrees F for 20 minutes.

4. Divide everything between plates and serve for lunch.

Nutrition Info: calories 322, fat 18.3, fiber 2, carbs 5.8, protein 35.7

Cheesy Stuffed Chicken_Ingredients:

2 scallions (meagerly cut)

2 seeded jalapeños (meagerly cut)

1/4 c. cilantro

1 tsp. lime pizzazz

4 oz. Monterey Jack cheddar (coarsely ground) 4 little boneless, skinless chicken bosoms

3 tbsp. olive oil

Salt

Pepper

3 tbsp. lime juice

2 ringer peppers (daintily cut)

1/2 little red onion (meagerly cut)

5 c. torn romaine lettuce

Directions:

1. Warmth broiler to 450°F. In bowl, consolidate scallions and seeded jalapeños, 1/4 cup cilantro (cleaved) and lime get-up-and-go, at that point hurl with Monterey Jack cheddar.

2. Supplement blade into thickest piece of every one of boneless, skinless chicken bosoms and move to and fro to make 2 1/2-inch pocket that is as wide as conceivable without experiencing. Stuff chicken with cheddar blend.

3. Warmth 2 tablespoons olive oil in enormous skillet on medium.

Season chicken with salt and pepper and cook until brilliant darker on 1 side, 3 to 4 minutes. Turn chicken over and broil until cooked through, 10 to 12 minutes.

4. In the interim, in huge bowl, whisk together lime juice, 1

tablespoon olive oil and 1/2 teaspoon salt. Include ringer peppers and red onion and let sit 10 minutes, hurling sporadically. Hurl with romaine lettuce and 1 cup new cilantro. Present with chicken and lime wedges.

Arugula With Gorgonzola Dressing *Servings: 4*

Cooking Time: 0 Minutes

Ingredients:

1 bunch of arugulas, cleaned

1 pear, sliced thinly

1 tablespoon fresh lemon juice

1 garlic clove, bruised

1/3 cup Gorgonzola cheese, crumbled

1/4 cup vegetable stock, reduced-sodium

Freshly ground pepper

4 teaspoons olive oil

1 tablespoon of cider vinegar

Directions:

1. Put the pear slices and lemon juice in a bowl. Toss to coat.

Arrange the pear slices, along with the arugula, on a platter.

2. In a bowl, combine the vinegar, oil, cheese, broth, pepper, and garlic. Leave for 5 minutes, remove the garlic. Put the dressing, then serve.

Nutrition Info: Calories 145 Carbs: 23g Fat: 4g Protein: 6g

Cabbage Soup *Servings: 6*

Cooking Time: 35 Minutes

Ingredients:

1 yellow onion, chopped

1 green cabbage head, shredded

2 tablespoons olive oil

5 cups veggie stock

1 carrot, peeled and grated

A pinch of salt and black pepper

1 tablespoon cilantro, chopped

2 teaspoons thyme, chopped

½ teaspoon smoked paprika

½ teaspoon hot paprika

1 tablespoon lemon juice

Cauliflower Rice _Servings: 4_

Cooking Time: 10 Minutes

Ingredients:

¼ cup Cooking Oil

1 tbsp. Coconut Oil

1 tbsp. Coconut Sugar

4 cups Cauliflower, broken down into florets ½ tsp. Salt

Directions:

1. First, process the cauliflower in a food processor and process it for 1 to 2 minutes.

2. Heat-up the oil in a large skillet over medium heat, then spoon in the riced cauliflower, coconut sugar, and salt to the pan.

3. Combine them well and cook them for 4 to 5 minutes or until the cauliflower is slightly soft.

4. Finally, pour the coconut milk and enjoy it.

Nutrition Info: Calories 108Kcal Proteins:27.1g Carbohydrates: 11g Fat: 6g

Feta Frittata & Spinach Servings: 4

Cooking Time: 10 Minutes

Ingredients:

½ small brown onion

250g baby spinach

½ cup feta cheese

1 tbsp garlic paste

4 beaten eggs

Seasoning Mix

Salt & Pepper according to taste

1 tbsp olive oil

Directions:

1. Add finely chop an onion in oil and cook it on medium flame.

2. Add spinach in light brown onions and toss it for 2 min.

3. In eggs, add the mixture of cold spinach and onions.

4. Now add garlic paste, salt, and pepper and mix the mixture.

5. Cook this mixture on low flame and stir eggs gently.

6. Add feta cheese on the eggs and place the pan under the already preheat grill.

7. Cook it almost for 2 to 3 minutes until the frittata is brown.

8. Serve this feta frittata hot or cold.

Nutrition Info: Calories 210 Carbs: 5g Fat: 14g Protein: 21g

Fiery Chicken Pot Stickers Ingredients:

1-pound ground chicken

1/2 cup destroyed cabbage

1 carrot, stripped and destroyed

2 cloves garlic, squeezed

2 green onions, meagerly cut

1 tablespoon diminished sodium soy sauce

1 tablespoon hoisin sauce

1 tablespoon naturally ground ginger

2 teaspoons sesame oil

1/4 teaspoon ground white pepper

36 won ton wrappers

2 tablespoons vegetable oil

FOR THE HOT CHILI OIL SAUCE:

1/2 cup vegetable oil

1/4 cup dried red chillies, squashed

2 cloves garlic, minced

Directions:

1. Warmth vegetable oil in a little pan over medium warmth. Mix in squashed peppers and garlic, mixing every so often, until the oil arrives at 180 degrees F, around 8-10 minutes; put in a safe spot.

2. In an enormous bowl, join chicken, cabbage, carrot, garlic, green onions, soy sauce, hoisin sauce, ginger, sesame oil and white pepper.

3. To collect the dumplings, place wrappers on a work surface.

Spoon 1 tablespoon of the chicken blend into the focal point of every wrapper. Utilizing your finger, rub the edges of the wrappers with water. Crease the mixture over the filling to make a half-moon shape, squeezing the edges to seal.

4. Warmth vegetable oil in a huge skillet over medium warmth.

Include pot stickers in a solitary layer and cook until brilliant and fresh, around 2-3 minutes for each side.

5. Serve promptly with hot stew oil sauce.

Garlic Shrimps With Gritted Cauliflower

Servings: 2

Cooking Time: 15 Minutes

Ingredients:

For Preparing Shrimps

1 Pound Shrimps

2-3tbsp Cajun seasoning

Salt

1tbsp Butter/Ghee

For Preparing Cauliflower Grits

2tbsp Ghee

12-Ounces of Cauliflower

1 Garlic clove

Salt-to-taste

Directions:

1. Boil cauliflower and garlic in 8ounces of water on medium flame until it's tender.

2. Blend tender cauliflower in the food processor with ghee. Add steaming water gradually for the right consistency.

3. Sprinkle 2tbsp of Cajun seasoning on shrimps and marinate.

4. In a large skillet, take 3tbsp of ghee and cook shrimps on medium flame.

5. Place a large spoon of cauliflower grits in bowl top up with fried shrimps.

Nutrition Info: Calories 107 Carbs: 1g Fat: 3g Protein: 20g

Broccoli Tuna _Servings: 1_

Cooking Time: 10 Minutes

Ingredients:

1 tsp. Extra Virgin Olive Oil

3oz. Tuna in water, preferably light & chunky, drained 1 tbsp. Walnuts, chopped coarsely

2 cups Broccoli, chopped finely

½ tsp. Hot Sauce

Directions:

1. Begin by mixing broccoli, seasoning & tuna in a large-sized mixing bowl until they are well combined.

2. Then, microwave the veggies in the oven for 3 minutes or until tender

3. Then, stir in the walnuts and olive oil to the bowl and mix well.

4. Serve and enjoy.

Nutrition Info: Calories 259Kcal Proteins:27.1g Carbohydrates: 12.9g Fat: 12.4g

Butternut Squash Soup With Shrimp _Servings: 4_

Cooking Time: 20 Minutes

Ingredients:

3 tablespoons unsalted butter

1 small red onion, finely chopped

1 garlic clove, sliced

1 teaspoon turmeric

1 teaspoon salt

¼ teaspoon freshly ground black pepper

3 cups vegetable broth

2 cups peeled butternut squash cut into ¼-inch dice 1-pound cooked peeled shrimp, thawed if necessary 1 cup unsweetened almond milk

¼ cup slivered almonds (optional)

2 tablespoons finely chopped fresh flat-leaf parsley 2 teaspoons grated or minced lemon zest

Directions:

1. Dissolve the butter over high heat in a large pot.

2. Add the onion, garlic, turmeric, salt, and pepper and sauté until the vegetables are soft and translucent, 5 to 7 minutes.

3. Add the broth and squash and boil.

4. Simmer within 5 minutes.

5. Add the shrimp and almond milk and cook until heated through about 2 minutes.

6. Sprinkle with the almonds (if using), parsley, and lemon zest and serve.

Nutrition Info: Calories 275 Total Fat: 12g Total Carbohydrates: 12g Sugar: 3g Fiber: 2g Protein: 30g Sodium: 1665mg

Tasty Turkey Baked Balls *Servings: 6*

Cooking Time: 30 Minutes

Ingredients:

1 pound ground turkey

½-cup fresh breadcrumbs, white or whole wheat ½-cup Parmesan cheese, freshly grated

½-Tbsp. basil, freshly chopped

½-Tbsp. oregano, freshly chopped

1-pc large egg, beaten

1-Tbsp. parsley, freshly chopped

3-Tbsp.s milk or water

A dash of salt and pepper

A pinch of freshly grated nutmeg

Directions:

1. Preheat your oven to 350°F.

2. Line two baking pans with parchment paper.

3. Stir in all of the ingredients in a large mixing bowl.

4. Form 1-inch balls from the mixture and place each ball in the baking pan.

5. Put the pan in the oven.

6. Bake for 30 minutes, or until the turkey cooks through and the surfaces turn brown.

7. Turn the meatballs once halfway into the cooking.

<u>Nutrition Info:</u> Calories: 517 CalFat: 17.2 g Protein: 38.7 g Carbs: 52.7 gFiber: 1 g

Clear Clam Chowder <u>*Servings: 4*</u>

Cooking Time: 15 Minutes

Ingredients:

2 tablespoons unsalted butter

2 medium carrots, cut into ½-inch pieces

2 celery stalks, thinly sliced

1 small red onion, cut into ¼-inch dice

2 garlic cloves, sliced

2 cups vegetable broth

1 (8-ounce) bottle clam juice

1 (10-ounce) can clams

½ teaspoon dried thyme

½ teaspoon salt

¼ teaspoon freshly ground black pepper

Directions:

1. Dissolve the butter in a large pot, over high heat.

2. Add the carrots, celery, onion, and garlic and sauté until slightly softened 2 to 3 minutes.

3. Add the broth and clam juice and boil.

4. Simmer and cook until the carrots are soft, 3 to 5 minutes.

5. Stir in the clams and their juices, thyme, salt, and pepper, heat through for 2 to 3 minutes, and serve.

Nutrition Info: Calories 156 Total Fat: 7g Total Carbohydrates: 7g Sugar: 3g Fiber: 1g Protein: 14g Sodium: 981mg

Rice And Chicken Pot Servings: 4

Cooking Time: 25 Minutes

Ingredients:

1 lb. free-range chicken breast, boneless, skinless ¼ cup of brown rice

¾ lb. mushrooms of choice, sliced

1 leek, chopped

¼ cup almonds, chopped

1 cup of water

1 Tbsp. olive oil

1 cup green beans

½ cup apple cider vinegar

2 Tbsp. all-purpose flour

1 cup milk, low fat

¼ cup Parmesan cheese, freshly grated

¼ cup sour cream

Pinch of sea salt, add more if needed

ground black pepper, to taste

Directions:

1. Pour brown rice into a pot. Add in water. Cover and bring to a boil. Lower the heat, then simmer for 30 minutes or until rice is cooked.

2. Meanwhile, in a skillet, add the chicken breast and pour just enough water to cover—season with salt. Boil the mixture, then reduce heat and allow to simmer for 10 minutes.

3. Shred the chicken. Set aside.

4. Warm the olive oil. Cook leeks until tender. Add in mushrooms.

5. Pour apple cider vinegar into the mixture. Sauté the mixture until the vinegar has evaporated. Add in flour and milk into the skillet.

Sprinkle Parmesan cheese and add in sour cream. Season with black pepper.

6. Preheat the oven to 350 degrees F. lightly grease a casserole dish with oil.

7. Spread cooked rice in the casserole dish, then the shredded chicken and green beans on top. Add mushrooms and leeks sauce.

Put almonds on top.

8. Bake within 20 minutes or until golden brown. Allow cooling before serving.

Nutrition Info: Calories 401 Carbs: 54g Fat: 12g Protein: 20g

Sautéed Shrimp Jambalaya Jumble Servings: 4

Cooking Time: 30 Minutes

Ingredients:

10-oz. medium shrimp, peeled

¼-cup celery, chopped ½-cup onion, chopped

1-Tbsp. oil or butter ¼-tsp garlic, minced

¼-tsp onion salt or sea salt

⅓-cup tomato sauce ½-tsp smoked paprika

½-tsp Worcestershire sauce

⅔-cup carrots, chopped

1¼-cups chicken sausage, precooked and diced 2-cups lentils, soaked overnight and precooked 2-cups okra, chopped

A dash of crushed red pepper and black pepper Parmesan cheese, grated for topping (optional) Directions:

1. Sauté the shrimp, celery, and onion with oil in a pan placed over medium-high heat for five minutes, or until the shrimp turn pinkish.

2. Add in the rest of the ingredients, and sauté further for 10

minutes, or until the veggies are tender.

3. To serve, divide the jambalaya mixture equally among four serving bowls.

4. Top with pepper and cheese, if desired.

Nutrition Info: Calories: 529Fat: 17.6gProtein: 26.4gCarbs: 98.4gFiber: 32.3g

Chicken Chili *Servings: 6*

Cooking Time: 1 Hour

Ingredients:

1 yellow onion, chopped

2 tablespoons olive oil

2 garlic cloves, minced

1-pound chicken breast, skinless, boneless and cubed 1 green bell pepper, chopped

2 cups chicken stock

1 tablespoon cocoa powder

2 tablespoons chili powder

1 teaspoon smoked paprika

1 cup canned tomatoes, chopped

1 tablespoon cilantro, chopped

A pinch of salt and black pepper

Directions:

1. Heat up a pot with the oil over medium heat, add the onion and the garlic and sauté for 5 minutes.

2. Add the meat and brown it for 5 minutes more.

3. Add the rest of the ingredients, toss, cook over medium heat for 40 minutes.

4. Divide the chili into bowls and serve for lunch.

Nutrition Info: calories 300, fat 2, fiber 10, carbs 15, protein 11

Garlic And Lentil Soup *Servings: 4*

Cooking Time: 15 Minutes

Ingredients:

2 tablespoons extra-virgin olive oil

2 medium carrots, thinly sliced

1 small white onion, cut into ¼-inch dice

2 garlic cloves, thinly sliced

1 teaspoon ground cinnamon

1 teaspoon salt

¼ teaspoon freshly ground black pepper

3 cups vegetable broth

1 (15-ounce) can lentils, drained and rinsed 1 tablespoon minced or grated orange zest

¼ cup chopped walnuts (optional)

2 tablespoons finely chopped fresh flat-leaf parsley Directions:

1. Heat-up the oil over high heat in a large pot.

2. Put the carrots, onion, and garlic and sauté until softened, 5 to 7 minutes.

3. Put the cinnamon, salt, and pepper and stir to coat the vegetables, 1 to 2 minutes evenly.

4. Put the broth and boil. Simmer, then put the lentils, and cook until within 1 minute.

5. Stir in the orange zest and serve, sprinkled with the walnuts (if using) and parsley.

<u>Nutrition Info:</u> Calories 201 Total Fat: 8g Total Carbohydrates: 22g Sugar: 4g Fiber: 8g Protein: 11g Sodium: 1178mg

Zesty Zucchini & Chicken In Classic Santa Fe Stir-fry

Servings: 2

Cooking Time: 15 Minutes

Ingredients:

1-Tbsp. olive oil

2-pcs chicken breasts, sliced

1-pc onion, small, diced

2-cloves garlic, minced 1-pc zucchini, diced ½- cup carrots, shredded

1-tsp paprika, smoked 1-tsp cumin, ground

½-tsp chili powder ¼-tsp sea salt

2-Tbsp. fresh lime juice

¼-cup cilantro, freshly chopped

Brown rice or quinoa, when serving

Directions:

1. Sauté the chicken with olive oil for about 3 minutes until the chicken turns brown. Set aside.

2. Use the same wok and add the onion and garlic.

3. Cook until the onion is tender.

4. Add in the carrots and zucchini.

5. Stir the mixture, and cook further for about a minute.

6. Add all the seasonings into the mix, and stir to cook for another minute.

7. Return the chicken in the wok, and pour in the lime juice.

8. Stir to cook until everything cooks through.

9. To serve, place the mixture over cooked rice or quinoa and top with the freshly chopped cilantro.

Nutrition Info: Calories: 191Fat: 5.3gProtein: 11.9gCarbs: 26.3gFiber: 2.5g

Tilapia Tacos With Awesome Ginger-sesame Slaw

Servings: 4

Cooking Time: 5 Hours

Ingredients:

1 tsp fresh ginger, grated

Salt and freshly cracked black pepper to taste 1 tsp stevia

1 tbsp soy sauce

1 tbsp olive oil

1 tbsp lemon juice

1 tbsp plain yogurt

1½lb tilapia fillets

1 cup coleslaw mix

Directions:

1. Switch on the instant pot, add all the ingredients in it, except for tilapia fillets and coleslaw mix, and stir until well combined.

2. Then add fillets, toss until well coated, shut with the lid, press the 'slow cook' button, and cook for 5 hours, flipping the fillets halfway through.

3. When done, transfer fillets to a dish and let cool completely.

4. For meal prep, distribute coleslaw mix between four air-tight containers, add tilapia and refrigerate for up to three days.

5. When ready to eat, reheat tilapia in the microwave until hot and then serve with coleslaw.

<u>Nutrition Info:</u> Calories 278, Total Fat 7.4g, Total Carbs 18.6g, Protein 35.9g, Sugar 1.2g, Fiber 8.2g, Sodium 194mg

Curry Lentil Stew *Servings: 4*

Cooking Time: 15 Minutes

Ingredients:

1 tablespoon of olive oil

1 onion, chopped

2 garlic cloves, minced

1 tablespoon of organic curry seasoning

4 cups of organic low-sodium vegetable broth 1 cup of red lentils

2 cups of butternut squash, cooked

1 cup of kale

1 teaspoon of turmeric

Sea salt to taste

Directions:

1. Sauté the olive oil with the onion and garlic in a large pot over medium heat, add. Sauté for 3 minutes.

2. Add in the organic curry seasoning, vegetable broth, and lentils, and bring to a boil—Cook for 10 minutes.

3. Stir in the cooked butternut squash and kale.

4. Add in the turmeric and sea salt to taste.

5. Serve warm.

<u>Nutrition Info:</u> Total Carbohydrates 41g Dietary Fiber: 13g Protein: 16g Total Fat: 4g Calories: 252

Kale Caesar Salad With Grilled Chicken Wrap

Servings: 2

Cooking Time: 20 Minutes

Ingredients:

6 cups curly kale, cut into small, bite-sized pieces ½ coddled egg; cooked

8 ounces grilled chicken, thinly sliced

½ teaspoon Dijon mustard

¾ cup Parmesan cheese, finely shredded

ground black pepper

kosher salt

1 garlic clove, minced

1 cup cherry tomatoes, quartered

1/8 cup lemon juice, freshly squeezed

2 large tortillas or two Lavash flatbreads

1 teaspoon agave or honey

1/8 cup olive oil

Directions:

1. Combine half of the coddled egg with mustard, minced garlic, honey, olive oil, and lemon juice in a large-sized mixing bowl. Whisk until you get dressing like consistency. Season with pepper and salt to taste.

2. Add the cherry tomatoes, chicken and kale; gently toss until nicely coated with the dressing & then add ¼ cup of parmesan.

3. Spread out the flatbreads & evenly distribute the prepared salad on top of the wraps; sprinkle each with approximately ¼ cup of the parmesan.

4. Roll up the wraps & slice into half. Serve immediately & enjoy.

Nutrition Info: kcal 511 Fat: 29 g Fiber: 2.8 g Protein: 50 g

Spinach Bean Salad *Servings: 1*

Cooking Time: 5 Minutes

Ingredients:

1 cup of fresh spinach

¼ cup of canned black beans

½ cup of canned garbanzo beans

½ cup of cremini mushrooms

2 tablespoons of organic balsamic vinaigrette 1 tablespoon of olive oil

Directions:

1. Cook the cremini mushrooms with the olive oil over low, medium heat for 5 minutes, until lightly browned.

2. Assemble the salad by adding the fresh spinach to a plate and topping it with the beans, mushrooms, and the balsamic vinaigrette.

Nutrition Info: Total Carbohydrates 26gg Dietary Fiber: 8g Protein: 9g Total Fat: 15g Calories: 274

Crusted Salmon With Walnuts & Rosemary

Servings: 6

Cooking Time: 20 Minutes

Ingredients:

1 Mince garlic clove

1tbsp Dijon mustard

¼ tbsp Lemon zest

1tbsp Lemon juice

1tbsp fresh rosemary

1/2 tbsp Honey

Olive oil

Fresh parsley

3tbsp Chopped walnuts

1 Pound skinless salmon

1tbsp Fresh crushed red pepper

Salt & pepper

Lemon wedges for garnish

3tbsp Panko breadcrumbs

1tbsp extra-virgin olive oil

Directions:

1. Spread the baking sheet in the oven and preheat it at 240C.

2. In a bowl, mix mustard paste, garlic, salt, olive oil, honey, lemon juice, crushed red pepper, rosemary, pus honey.

3. Combine panko, walnuts, and oil and spread thin fish slice on the baking sheet. Spray olive oil equally on both sides of the fish.

4. Place walnut mixture on the salmon with the mustard mixture on top it.

5. Bake the salmon almost for 12 minutes. Garnish it with fresh parsley and lemon wedges and serve it hot.

Nutrition Info: Calories 227 Carbs: 0g Fat: 12g Protein: 29g

Baked Sweet Potato With Red Tahini Sauce

Servings: 4

Cooking Time: 30 Minutes

Ingredients:

15-ounces Canned Chickpeas

4 Medium-sized sweet potatoes

½ tbsp Olive oil

1 Pinch salt

1tbsp Lime juice

1/2 tbsp of cumin, coriander, and paprika powder For Garlic Herb Sauce

¼ Cup tahini sauce

½ tbsp Lime Juice

3 cloves garlic

Salt to taste

Directions:

1. Preheat the oven at 204°C. Toss chickpeas in salt, spices & olive oil. Spread them on the foil sheet.

2. Brush sweet potato thin wedges with oil and place them on marinated beans and bake.

3. For the sauce, mix all fixings in a bowl. Add some water in it, but keep it thick.

4. Remove sweet potatoes from the oven after 25 minutes.

5. Garnish this baked sweet potato chickpea salad with hot garlic sauce.

Nutrition Info: Calories 90 Carbs: 20g Fat: 0g Protein: 2g

Italian Summer Squash Soup *Servings: 4*

Cooking Time: 15 Minutes

Ingredients:

3 tablespoons extra-virgin olive oil

1 small red onion, thinly sliced

1 garlic clove, minced

1 cup shredded zucchini

1 cup shredded yellow squash

½ cup shredded carrot

3 cups vegetable broth

1 teaspoon salt

2 tablespoons finely chopped fresh basil

1 tablespoon finely chopped fresh chives

2 tablespoons pine nuts

Directions:

1. Heat-up the oil over high heat in a large pot.

2. Put the onion and garlic and sauté until softened, 5 to 7 minutes.

3. Add the zucchini, yellow squash, and carrot and sauté until softened, 1 to 2 minutes.

4. Add the broth and salt, and boil. Simmer within 1 to 2 minutes.

5. Stir in the basil and chives and serve, sprinkled with the pine nuts.

<u>Nutrition Info:</u> Calories 172 Total Fat: 15g Total Carbohydrates: 6g Sugar: 3g Fiber: 2g Protein: 5g Sodium: 1170mg

Saffron And Salmon Soup Servings: 4

Cooking Time: 20 Minutes

Ingredients:

¼ cup extra-virgin olive oil

2 leeks, white parts only, thinly sliced

2 medium carrots, thinly sliced

2 garlic cloves, thinly sliced

4 cups vegetable broth

1-pound skinless salmon fillets, cut into 1-inch pieces 1 teaspoon salt

¼ teaspoon freshly ground black pepper

¼ teaspoon saffron threads

2 cups baby spinach

½ cup dry white wine

2 tablespoons chopped scallions, both white and green parts 2 tablespoons finely chopped fresh flat-leaf parsley Directions:

1. Heat the oil over high in a large pot.

2. Add the leeks, carrots, and garlic and sauté until softened, 5 to 7 minutes.

3. Put the broth and boil.

4. Simmer and add the salmon, salt, pepper, and saffron. Cook until the salmon is cooked through, about 8 minutes.

5. Add the spinach, wine, scallions, and parsley and cook until the spinach has wilted, 1 to 2 minutes, and serve.

Nutrition Info: Calories 418 Total Fat: 26g Total Carbohydrates: 13g Sugar: 4g Fiber: 2g Protein: 29g Sodium: 1455mg

Thai Flavored Hot And Sour Shrimp And Mushroom Soup

Servings: 6

Cooking Time: 38 Minutes

Ingredients:

3 tbsp unsalted butter

1lb shrimp, peeled and deveined

2 tsp minced garlic

1-inch piece ginger root, peeled

1 medium onion, diced

1 red Thai chili, chopped

1 lemongrass stalk

½ tsp fresh lime zest

Salt and freshly cracked black pepper, to taste 5 cups chicken broth

1 tbsp coconut oil

½lb cremini mushrooms, sliced into wedges

1 small green zucchini

2 tbsp fresh lime juice

2 tbsp fish sauce

¼ bunch of fresh Thai basil, chopped

¼ bunch of fresh cilantro, chopped

Directions:

1. Take a large pot, place it over medium heat, add butter and when it melts, add shrimps, garlic, ginger, onion, chilies, lemongrass, and lime zest, season with salt and black pepper and cook for 3 minutes.

2. Pour in broth, simmer for 30 minutes, and then strain it.

3. Take a large skillet pan over medium heat, add oil and when hot, add mushrooms and zucchini, season more with salt and black pepper and cook for 3 minutes.

4. Add shrimp's mixture in the skillet pan, simmer for 2 minutes, drizzle with lime juice and fish sauce and cook for 1 minute.

5. Taste to adjust seasoning, then remove the pan from heat, garnish with cilantro and basil and serve.

Nutrition Info: Calories 223, Total Fat 10.2g, Total Carbs 8.7g, Protein 23g, Sugar 3.6g, Sodium 1128mg

Orzo With Sundried Tomatoes Ingredients:

1 lb boneless skinless chicken bosoms, diced into 3/4-inch pieces

1 Tbsp + 1 tsp olive oil

Salt and crisply ground dark pepper

2 cloves garlic, minced

1/4 cups (8 oz) dry orzo pasta

2 3/4 cups low-sodium chicken stock, at that point more varying (don't utilize ordinary juices, it will be excessively salty) 1/3 cup sun dried tomato parts stuffed in oil with herbs (around 12 parts. Shake off a portion of the abundance oil), hacked fine in a nourishment processor

1/2 - 3/4 cup finely destroyed parmesan cheddar, to taste 1/3 cup cleaved crisp basil

Directions:

1. Warmth 1 Tbsp olive oil in a saute container over medium-high warmth.

2. Once gleaming include chicken, season gently with salt and pepper and cook until brilliant, around 3 minutes at that point pivot to inverse sides and cook until brilliant dark colored and cooked through, around 3 minutes. Move chicken to a plate, spread with foil to keep warm.

3. Include staying 1 tsp olive oil to saute dish at that point include garlic and saute 20 seconds, or just until daintily brilliant, at that point pour in chicken juices while scraping up cooked bits from base of skillet.

4. Heat stock to the point of boiling at that point include orzo pasta, lessen warmth to medium spread skillet with cover and permit to delicately bubble 5 minutes at that point reveal, mix and keep on bubbling revealed until orzo is delicate, around 5 minutes longer, blending at times (don't stress if there's still a little juices, it will give it some saucy-ness).

5. When pasta has cooked through hurl chicken in with orzo at that point expel from heat. Include parmesan cheddar and mix until dissolved, at that point hurl in sun dried tomatoes, basil and season

with pepper (you shouldn't require any salt however include a little in the event that you'd think it needs it).

6. Add more juices to thin whenever wanted (as the pasta rests it will absorb abundance fluid and I enjoyed it with somewhat overabundance so I included somewhat more). Serve warm.

Mushroom And Beet Soup _Servings: 4_

Cooking Time: 40 Minutes

Ingredients:

2 tablespoons olive oil

1 yellow onion, chopped

2 beets, peeled and cut into large cubes

1-pound white mushrooms, sliced

2 garlic cloves, minced

1 tablespoon tomato paste

5 cups veggie stock

1 tablespoons parsley, chopped

Directions:

1. Heat up a pot with the oil over medium heat, add the onion and the garlic and sauté for 5 minutes.

2. Add the mushrooms, stir and sauté for 5 minutes more.

3. Add the beets and the other ingredients, bring to a simmer and cook over medium heat for 30 minutes more, stirring from time to time.

4. Ladle the soup into bowls and serve.

Nutrition Info: calories 300, fat 5, fiber 9, carbs 8, protein 7

Chicken Parmesan Meatballs Ingredients:

2 pounds ground chicken

3/4 cup panko breadcrumbs gluten free panko will work fine 1/4 cup finely minced onion

2 tablespoons minced parsley

2 cloves garlic minced

get-up-and-go of 1 little lemon around 1 teaspoon 2 eggs

3/4 cup destroyed Pecorino Romano or Parmesan cheddar 1 teaspoon genuine salt

1/2 teaspoon crisply ground dark pepper

1 quart Five Minute Marinara Sauce

4-6 ounces mozzarella crisply cut

Directions:

1. Preheat the stove to 400 degrees, setting the rack in the upper third of the broiler. In a huge bowl, join everything aside from the marinara and the mozzarella. Softly combine, utilizing your hands or an enormous spoon. Scoop and shape into little meatballs and spot on a foil lined heating sheet. Spot the meatballs genuinely near one another on the plate to make them

fit. Spoon about a half tablespoon of sauce over every meatball. Heat for 15 minutes.

2. Expel meatballs from the stove and increment the broiler temperature to cook. Spoon an extra half tablespoon of sauce over every meatball and top with a little square of mozzarella. (I cut the slight cuts into pieces around 1" square.) Broil an extra 3 minutes, until the cheddar has softened and turned brilliant. Present with extra sauce. Appreciate!

Meatballs Alla Parmigiana Ingredients:

For the meatballs

1.5lbs ground hamburger (80/20)

2 Tbl crisp parsley, cleaved

3/4 cup ground parmesan cheddar

1/2 cup almond flour

2 eggs

1 tsp fit salt

1/4 tsp ground dark pepper

1/4 tsp garlic powder

1 tsp dried onion drops

1/4 tsp dried oregano

1/2 cup warm water

For the Parmigiana

1 cup simple keto marinara sauce (or any sugar free locally acquired marinara)

4 oz mozzarella cheddar

Directions:

1. Join the entirety of the meatball fixings in a huge bowl and blend well.

2. Structure into fifteen 2" meatballs.

3. Prepare at 350 degrees (F) for 20 minutes OR fry in an enormous skillet over medium warmth until cooked through. Ace tip – have a go at searing in bacon oil in the event that you have any – it includes another degree of flavor. Fricasseeing produces the brilliant dark colored shading appeared in the photographs above.

4. For the Parmigiana:

5. Spot the cooked meatballs in a stove safe dish.

6. Spoon roughly 1 Tbl sauce over every meatball.

7. Spread with roughly 1/4 oz of mozzarella cheddar each.

8. Prepare at 350 degrees (F) for 20 minutes (40 minutes if meatballs are solidified) or until warmed through and the cheddar is brilliant.

9. Embellishment with new parsley whenever wanted.

Sheet Pan Turkey Breast With Golden Vegetables

Servings: 4

Cooking Time: 45 Minutes

Ingredients:

2 tablespoons unsalted butter, at room temperature 1 medium acorn squash, seeded and thinly sliced 2 large golden beets, peeled and thinly sliced ½ medium yellow onion, thinly sliced

½ boneless, skin-on turkey breast (1 to 2 pounds) 2 tablespoons honey

1 teaspoon salt

1 teaspoon turmeric

¼ teaspoon freshly ground black pepper

1 cup chicken broth or vegetable broth

Directions:

1. Preheat the oven to 400°F. Grease the baking sheet with the butter.

2. Arrange the squash, beets, and onion in a single layer on the baking sheet. Put the turkey skin-side up. Drizzle with the honey.

Season with the salt, turmeric, and pepper, and add the broth.

3. Roast until the turkey registers 165°F in the center with an instant-read thermometer, 35 to 45 minutes. Remove, and let rest for 5 minutes.

4. Slice, and serve.

Nutrition Info: Calories 383 Total Fat: 15g Total Carbohydrates: 25g Sugar: 13g Fiber: 3g Protein: 37g Sodium: 748mg

Coconut Green Curry With Boil Rice *Servings: 8*

Cooking Time: 20 Minutes

Ingredients:

2tbsp Olive oil

12ounces of Tofu

2 medium sweet potatoes (cut into cubes)

Salt-to-taste

314ounces Coconut milk

4tbsp Green curry paste

3 Cups of Broccoli Florets

Directions:

1. Remove excess water from tofu and fry it on medium flame. Add salt in it and fry it for 12 minutes.

2. Cook coconut milk, green curry paste, and sweet potato on medium heat and simmer it for 5 mins.

3. Now add broccoli and tofu in it and cook it almost 5 minutes until the broccoli color changes.

4. Serve this coconut and green curry with a handful of boil rice and many raisins on top of it.

Nutrition Info: Calories 170 Carbs: 34g Fat: 2g Protein: 3g

Sweet Potato & Chicken Soup With Lentil

Servings: 6

Cooking Time: 35 Minutes

Ingredients:

10 Celery stalks

1 Home-cooked or rotisserie chicken

2 medium sweet potatoes

5-ounces French lentils

2tbsp Fresh lime juice

½ head bite-size escarole

6 thin-sliced garlic cloves

½ Cup dill (finely chop)

1tbsp Kosher Salt

2tbsp Extra virgin oil

Directions:

1. Add salt, chicken carcass, lentil, and sweet potatoes in 8 ounces of water and boil it on high flame.

2. Cook these items almost for 10-12 minutes and skim off all the foam form on it.

3. Cook garlic and celery in oil almost for 10 minutes until it is tender

& light brown, then add shredded roast chicken in it.

4. Add this mixture in the escarole soup and continuously stir it for 5

minutes on medium heat.

5. Add lemon juice and stir in dill. Serve season hot soup with salt.

Nutrition Info: Calories 310 Carbs: 45g Fat: 11g Protein: 13g

Creamy Pork And Tomatoes Servings: 4

Cooking Time: 35 Minutes

Ingredients:

2 pounds pork stew meat, cubed

2 tablespoons avocado oil

1 cup tomatoes, cubed

1 cup coconut cream

1 tablespoon mint, chopped

1 jalapeno pepper, chopped

A pinch of sea salt and black pepper

1 tablespoon hot pepper

2 tablespoons lemon juice

Directions:

1. Heat up a pan with the oil over medium heat, add the meat and brown for 5 minutes.

2. Add the rest of the ingredients, toss, cook over medium heat for 30 minutes more, divide between plates and serve.

Nutrition Info: calories 230, fat 4, fiber 6, carbs 9, protein 14

Lemon Tenderloin _Servings: 2_

Cooking Time: 25 Minutes

Ingredients:

¼ teaspoon za'atar seasoning

Zest of 1 lemon

½ teaspoon dried thyme

¼ teaspoon garlic powder

¼ teaspoon salt

1 tablespoon olive oil

1 (8-ounce / 227-g) pork tenderloin, sliver skin trimmed Directions:

1. Preheat the oven to 425ºF (220ºC).

2. Combine the za'atar seasoning, lemon zest, thyme, garlic powder, and salt in a bowl, then rub the pork tenderloin with the mixture on both sides.

3. Warm the olive oil in an oven-safe skillet over medium-high heat until shimmering.

4. Add the pork tenderloin and sear for 6 minutes or until browned.

Flip the pork halfway through the cooking time.

5. Arrange the skillet in the preheated oven and roast for 15 minutes or until an instant-read thermometer inserted in the thickest part of the tenderloin registers at least 145ºF (63ºC).

6. Transfer the cooked tenderloin to a large plate and allow to cool for a few minutes before serving.

Nutrition Info: calories: 184 ; fat: 10.8g ; carbs: 1.2g ; fiber: 0g ; protein: 20.1g ; sodium: 358mg

Chicken With Broccoli _Servings: 4_

Ingredients:

1 chopped small white onion

1½ c. low-fat, low-sodium chicken broth

Freshly ground black pepper

2 c. chopped broccoli

1 lb. cubed, skinless and de-boned chicken thighs 2 minced garlic cloves

Directions:

1. In a slow cooker, add all ingredients and mix well.

2. Set slow cooker on low.

3. Cover and cook for 4-5 hours.

4. Serve hot.

Nutrition Info: Calories: 300, Fat:9 g, Carbs:19 g, Protein:31 g, Sugars:6 g, Sodium:200 mg

Crispy Chicken Tenderloin Servings: 4

Cooking Time: 15 Minutes

Ingredients:

1 egg, beaten

8 chicken tenderloin

2 tablespoons avocado oil

½ cup breadcrumbs

Directions:

1. Preheat your air fryer to 350 degrees F.

2. Dip chicken in egg.

3. Mix oil and breadcrumbs.

4. Coat chicken with this mixture.

5. Add to the air fryer basket.

6. Cook for 15 minutes.

Pork With Mushrooms And Cucumbers

Servings: 4

Cooking Time: 25 Minutes

Ingredients:

2 tablespoons olive oil

½ teaspoon oregano, dried

4 pork chops

2 garlic cloves, minced

Juice of 1 lime

¼ cup cilantro, chopped

A pinch of sea salt and black pepper

1 cup white mushrooms, halved

2 tablespoons balsamic vinegar

Directions:

1. Heat up a pan with the oil over medium heat, add the pork chops and brown for 2 minutes on each side.

2. Add the rest of the ingredients, toss, cook over medium heat for 20 minutes, divide between plates and serve.

Nutrition Info: calories 220, fat 6, fiber 8, carbs 14.2, protein 20

Chicken Chopstick _Servings: 4_

Ingredients:

¼ c. diced chopped onion

1 pack cooked chow Mein noodles

Fresh ground pepper

2 cans cream mushroom soup

1 ¼ c. sliced celery

1 c. cashew nuts

2 c. cubed cooked chicken

½ c. water

Directions:

1. Preheat the oven to 375°F.

2. In a pot suitable for the oven, pour in both cans of cream of mushroom soup and water. Mix until combined.

3. Add the cooked cubed chicken, onion, celery, pepper, cashew nuts to the soup. Stir until combined. Add half the noodles to the mixture, stir until coated.

4. Top the casserole with the rest of the noodles.

5. Place the pot in the oven. Bake for 25 minutes.

6. Serve immediately.

Nutrition Info: Calories: 201, Fat:17 g, Carbs:15 g, Protein:13 g, Sugars:7 g, Sodium:10 mg

Balsamic Roast Chicken Servings: 4

Ingredients:

1 tbsp. minced fresh rosemary

1 minced garlic clove

Black pepper

1 tbsp. olive oil

1 tsp. brown sugar

6 rosemary sprigs

1 whole chicken

½ c. balsamic vinegar

Directions:

1. Combine garlic, minced rosemary, black pepper and the olive oil. Rub the chicken with the herbal olive oil mixture.

2. Put 3 rosemary sprigs into the chicken cavity.

3. Place the chicken into a roasting pan and roast at 400F for about 1 hr. 30 minutes.

4. When the chicken is golden and the juices run clear, transfer to a serving dish.

5. In a saucepan dissolve the sugar in balsamic vinegar over heat. Do not boil.

6. Carve the chicken and top with vinegar mixture.

Nutrition Info: Calories: 587, Fat:37.8 g, Carbs:2.5 g, Protein:54.1 g, Sugars:0 g, Sodium:600 mg

Steak & Mushrooms _Servings: 4_

Cooking Time: 15 Minutes

Ingredients:

2 tablespoons olive oil

8 oz. mushrooms, sliced

½ teaspoon garlic powder

1 lb. steak, sliced into cubes

1 teaspoon (5 ml) Worcestershire sauce

Pepper to taste

Directions:

1. Preheat your air fryer to 400 degrees F.

2. Combine all ingredients in a bowl.

3. Transfer to the air fryer basket.

4. Cook for 15 minutes, shaking the basket twice.

Beef Tips Servings: 4

Cooking Time: 12 Minutes

Ingredients:

2 teaspoons onion powder

1 teaspoon garlic powder

2 teaspoons rosemary, chopped

1 teaspoon paprika

2 tablespoons low-sodium coconut amino

Pepper to taste

1 lb. steak, sliced into strips

Directions:

1. Mix all spices and seasoning in a bowl.

2. Stir in steak strips.

3. Marinate for 10 minutes.

4. Add to the air fryer basket.

5. Cook at 380 degrees F for 12 minutes, shaking once or twice halfway through the cooking.

Peach Chicken Treat Servings: 4-5

Ingredients:

2 minced garlic cloves

¼ c. balsamic vinegar

4 sliced peaches

4 skinless, deboned chicken breasts

¼ c. chopped basil

1 tbsp. olive oil

1 chopped shallot

¼ tsp. black pepper

Directions:

1. Heat up the oil in a saucepan over medium-high flame.

2. Add the meat and season with black pepper; fry for 8 minutes on each side and set aside to rest in a plate.

3. In the same pan, add the shallot and garlic; stir and cook for 2 minutes.

4. Add the peaches; stir and cook for 4-5 more minutes.

5. Add the vinegar, cooked chicken, and basil; toss and simmer covered for 3-4 minutes more.

6. Serve warm.

Nutrition Info: Calories: 270, Fat:0 g, Carbs:6.6 g, Protein:1.5 g, Sugars:24 g, Sodium:87 mg

Ground Pork Pan Servings: 4

Cooking Time: 15 Minutes

Ingredients:

2 garlic cloves, minced

2 red chilies, chopped

2 tablespoons olive oil

2 pounds pork stew meat, ground

1 red bell pepper, chopped

1 green bell pepper, chopped

1 tomato, cubed

½ cup mushrooms, halved

A pinch of sea salt and black pepper

1 tablespoon basil, chopped

2 tablespoons coconut aminos

Directions:

1. Heat up a pan with the oil over medium heat, add the garlic, chilies, bell peppers, tomato and the mushrooms and sauté for 5 minutes.

2. Add the meat and the rest of the ingredients, toss, cook over medium heat for 10 minutes more, divide between plates and serve.

Nutrition Info: calories 200, fat 3, fiber 5, carbs 7, protein 17

Parsley Pork And Artichokes *Servings: 4*

Cooking Time: 35 Minutes

Ingredients:

2 tablespoons balsamic vinegar

1 cup canned artichoke hearts, drained and quartered 2 tablespoons olive oil

2 pounds pork stew meat, cubed

2 tablespoons parsley, chopped

1 teaspoon cumin, ground

1 teaspoon turmeric powder

2 garlic cloves, minced

A pinch of sea salt and black pepper

Directions:

1. Heat up a pan with the oil over medium heat, add the meat and brown for 5 minutes.

2. Add the artichokes, the vinegar and the other ingredients, toss, cook over medium heat for 30 minutes, divide between plates and serve.

Nutrition Info: calories 260, fat 5, fiber 4, carbs 11, protein 20

Pork With Thyme Sweet Potatoes Servings: 4

Cooking Time: 35 Minutes

Ingredients:

2 sweet potatoes, peeled and cut into wedges 4 pork chops

3 spring onions, chopped

1 tablespoon thyme, chopped

2 tablespoons olive oil

4 garlic cloves, minced

A pinch of sea salt and black pepper

½ cup vegetable stock

½ tablespoon chives, chopped

Directions:

1. In a roasting pan, combine the pork chops with the potatoes and the other ingredients, toss gently and cook at 390 degrees F for 35 minutes.

2. Divide everything between plates and serve.

Nutrition Info: calories 210, fat 12.2, fiber 5.2, carbs 12, protein 10

Curry Pork Mix *Servings: 4*

Cooking Time: 30 Minutes

Ingredients:

2 tablespoon olive oil

4 scallions, chopped

2 garlic cloves, minced

2 pounds pork stew meat, cubed

2 tablespoons red curry paste

1 teaspoon chili paste

2 tablespoons balsamic vinegar

¼ cup vegetable stock

¼ cup parsley, chopped

Directions:

1. Heat up a pan with the oil over medium-high heat, add the scallions and the garlic and sauté for 5 minutes.

2. Add the meat and brown for 5 minutes more.

3. Add the remaining ingredients, toss, cook over medium heat for 20 minutes, divide between plates and serve.

Nutrition Info: calories 220, fat 3, fiber 4, carbs 7, protein 12

Stir-fried Chicken And Broccoli *Servings: 4*

Cooking Time: 10 Minutes

Ingredients:

3 tablespoons extra-virgin olive oil

1½ cups broccoli florets

1½ pounds (680 g) boneless, skinless chicken breasts, cut into bite-size pieces

½ onion, chopped

½ teaspoon sea salt

⅛ teaspoon freshly ground black pepper

3 garlic cloves, minced

2 cups cooked brown rice

Directions:

1. Heat the olive oil in a large nonstick skillet over medium-high heat until shimmering.

2. Add the broccoli, chicken, and onion to the skillet and stir well.

Season with sea salt and black pepper.

3. Stir-fry for about 8 minutes, or until the chicken is golden browned and cooked through.

4. Toss in the garlic and cook for 30 seconds, stirring constantly, or until the garlic is fragrant.

5. Remove from the heat to a plate and serve over the cooked brown rice.

Nutrition Info: calories: 344 ; fat: 14.1g ; protein: 14.1g ; carbs: 40.9g ; fiber: 3.2g ; sugar: 1.2g ; sodium: 275mg

Chicken And Broccoli Servings: 4

Ingredients:

2 minced garlic cloves

4 de-boned, skinless chicken breasts

½ c. coconut cream

1 tbsp. chopped oregano

2 c. broccoli florets

1 tbsp. organic olive oil

1 c. chopped red onions

Directions:

1. Heat up a pan while using the oil over medium-high heat, add chicken breasts and cook for 5 minutes on each side.

2. Add onions and garlic, stir and cook for 5 minutes more.

3. Add oregano, broccoli and cream, toss everything, cook for ten minutes more, divide between plates and serve.

4. Enjoy!

Nutrition Info: Calories: 287, Fat:10 g, Carbs:14 g, Protein:19 g, Sugars:10 g, Sodium:1106 mg

Mediterranean Chicken Bake With Vegetables

Servings: 4

Cooking Time: 20 Minutes

Ingredients:

4 (4-ounce / 113-g) boneless, skinless chicken breasts 2 tablespoons avocado oil

1 cup sliced cremini mushrooms

1 cup packed chopped fresh spinach

1 pint cherry tomatoes, halved

½ cup chopped fresh basil

½ red onion, thinly sliced

4 garlic cloves, minced

2 teaspoons balsamic vinegar

Directions:

1. Preheat the oven to 400ºF (205ºC).

2. Arrange the chicken breast in a large baking dish and brush them generously with the avocado oil.

3. Mix together the mushrooms, spinach, tomatoes, basil, red onion, cloves, and vinegar in a medium bowl, and toss to combine. Scatter each chicken breast with ¼ of the vegetable mixture.

4. Bake in the preheated oven for about 20 minutes, or until the internal temperature reaches at least 165ºF (74ºC) and juices run clear when pierced with a fork.

5. Allow the chicken to rest for 5 to 10 minutes before slicing to serve.

Nutrition Info: calories: 220 ; fat: 9.1g ; protein: 28.2g ; carbs: 6.9g ; fiber: 2.1g ; sugar: 6.7g ; sodium: 310mg

Hidden Valley Chicken Drummies Servings: 6 - 8

Ingredients:

2 tbsps. Hot sauce

½ c. melted butter

Celery sticks

2 packages Hidden Valley dressing dry mix

3 tbsps. Vinegar

12 chicken drumsticks

Paprika

Directions:

1. Preheat the oven to 350 0F.

2. Rinse and pat dry the chicken.

3. In a bowl blend the dry dressing, melted butter, vinegar and hot sauce. Stir until combined.

4. Place the drumsticks in a large plastic baggie, pour the sauce over drumsticks. Massage the sauce until the drumsticks are coated.

5. Place the chicken in a single layer on a baking dish. Sprinkle with paprika.

6. Bake for 30 minutes, flipping halfway.

7. Serve with crudité or salad.

Nutrition Info: Calories: 155, Fat:18 g, Carbs:96 g, Protein:15 g, Sugars:0.7 g, Sodium:340 mg

Balsamic Chicken And Beans *Servings: 4*

Ingredients:

1 lb. trimmed fresh green beans

¼ c. balsamic vinegar

2 sliced shallots

2 tbsps. Red pepper flakes

4 skinless, de-boned chicken breasts

2 minced garlic cloves

3 tbsps. Extra virgin olive oil

Directions:

1. Combine 2 tablespoons of the olive oil with the balsamic vinegar, garlic, and shallots. Pour it over the chicken breasts and refrigerate overnight.

2. The next day, preheat the oven to 375 OF.

3. Take the chicken out of the marinade and arrange in a shallow baking pan. Discard the rest of the marinade.

4. Bake in the oven for 40 minutes.

5. While the chicken is cooking, bring a large pot of water to a boil.

6. Place the green beans in the water and allow them to cook for five minutes and then drain.

7. Heat one tablespoon of olive oil in the pot and return the green beans after rinsing them.

8. Toss with red pepper flakes.

Nutrition Info: Calories: 433, Fat:17.4 g, Carbs:12.9 g, Protein:56.1 g, Sugars:13 g, Sodium:292 mg

Italian Pork Servings: 6

Cooking Time: 1 Hour

Ingredients:

2 pounds pork roast

3 tablespoons olive oil

2 teaspoons oregano, dried

1 tablespoon Italian seasoning

1 teaspoon rosemary, dried

1 teaspoon basil, dried

3 garlic cloves, minced

¼ cup vegetable stock

A pinch of salt and black pepper

Directions:

1. In a baking pan, combine the pork roast with the oil, the oregano and the other ingredients, toss and bake at 390 degrees F for 1 hour.

2. Slice the roast, divide it and the other ingredients between plates and serve.

Nutrition Info: calories 580, fat 33.6, fiber 0.5, carbs 2.3, protein 64.9

Chicken And Brussels Sprouts Servings: 4

Ingredients:

1 cored, peeled and chopped apple

1 chopped yellow onion

1 tbsp. organic olive oil

3 c. shredded Brussels sprouts

1 lb. ground chicken meat

Black pepper

Directions:

1. Heat up a pan while using oil over medium-high heat, add chicken, stir and brown for 5 minutes.

2. Add Brussels sprouts, onion, black pepper and apple, stir, cook for 10 minutes, divide into bowls and serve.

3. Enjoy!

Nutrition Info: Calories: 200, Fat:8 g, Carbs:13 g, Protein:9 g, Sugars:3.3 g, Sodium:194 mg

Chicken Divan Ingredients:

1 c. croutons

1 c. cooked and diced broccoli pieces

½ c. water

1 c. grated extra sharp cheddar cheese

½ lb. de-boned and skinless cooked chicken pieces 1 can mushroom soup

Directions:

1. Preheat the oven to 350°F

2. In a large pot, heat the soup and water. Add the chicken, broccoli, and cheese. Combine thoroughly.

3. Pour into a greased baking dish.

4. Place the croutons over the mixture.

5. Bake for 30 minutes or until the casserole is bubbling and the croutons are golden brown.

Nutrition Info: Calories: 380, Fat:22 g, Carbs:10 g, Protein:25 g, Sugars:2 g, Sodium:475 mg

Parmesan Chicken _Servings: 4_

Cooking Time: 10 Minutes

Ingredients:

4 chicken breast fillets

2 teaspoons garlic powder

2 teaspoons Italian seasoning

Pepper to taste

¼ cup Parmesan cheese

½ cup breadcrumbs

1 cup breadcrumbs

2 eggs, beaten

Cooking spray

Directions:

1. Flatten chicken breast with meat mallet.

2. Season with garlic powder, Italian seasoning and pepper.

3. Mix almond flour and Parmesan cheese in a bowl.

4. Add eggs to another bowl.

5. Dip chicken fillet in the eggs and then in the flour.

6. Spray with oil.

7. Place in the air fryer.

8. Cook at 350 degrees F for 10 minutes per side.

Sumptuous Indian Chicken Curry *Servings: 6*

Cooking Time: 20 Minutes

Ingredients:

2 tablespoons coconut oil, divided

2 (4-ounce / 113-g) boneless, skinless chicken breasts, cut into bite-size pieces

2 medium carrots, diced

1 small white onion, diced

1 tablespoon minced fresh ginger

6 garlic cloves, minced

1 cup sugar snap peas, diced

1 (5.4-ounce / 153-g) can unsweetened coconut cream 1 tablespoon sugar-free fish sauce

1 cup low-sodium chicken broth

½ cup diced tomatoes, with juice

1 tablespoon curry powder

¼ teaspoon sea salt

Pinch cayenne pepper, to taste

Freshly ground black pepper, to taste

¼ cup filtered water

Directions:

1. Heat 1 tablespoon of coconut oil in a nonstick skillet over medium-high heat until melted.

2. Add the chicken breasts to the skillet and cook for 15 minutes or until an instant-read thermometer inserted in the thickest part of the chicken breasts registers at least 165ºF (74ºC). Flip the chicken breasts halfway through the cooking time.

3. Meanwhile, in a separate skillet, heat the remaining coconut oil over medium heat until melted.

4. Add the carrots, onion, ginger, and garlic to the skillet and sauté for 5 minutes or until fragrant and the onion is translucent.

5. Add the peas, coconut cream, fish sauce, chicken broth, tomatoes, curry powder, salt, cayenne pepper, black pepper, and water to the skillet. Stir to mix well.

6. Bring to a boil. Reduce the heat to medium-low then simmer for 10 minutes.

7. Add the cooked chicken to the second skillet, then cook for 2

more minutes to combine well.

8. Pour the curry on a large serving plate, then serve immediately.

Nutrition Info: calories: 223 ; fat: 15.7g ; protein: 13.4g ; carbs: 9.4g

; fiber: 3.0g ; sugar: 2.3g ; sodium: 673mg

Pork With Balsamic Onion Sauce Servings: 4

Cooking Time: 35 Minutes

Ingredients:

1 yellow onion, chopped

4 scallions, chopped

2 tablespoons avocado oil

1 tablespoon rosemary, chopped

1 tablespoon lemon zest, grated

2 pounds pork roast, sliced

2 tablespoons balsamic vinegar

½ cup vegetable stock

A pinch of sea salt and black pepper

Directions:

1. Heat up a pan with the oil over medium heat, add the onion and the scallions and sauté for 5 minutes.

2. Add the rest of the ingredients except the meat, stir, and simmer for 5 minutes.

3. Add the meat, toss gently, cook over medium heat for 25 minutes, divide between plates and serve.

Nutrition Info: calories 217, fat 11, fiber 1, carbs 6, protein 14

373. Meatloaf Servings: 4

Cooking Time: 30 Minutes

Ingredients:

1 lb. lean ground beef

3 tablespoons breadcrumbs

1 onion, chopped

1 tablespoon fresh thyme, chopped

Garlic powder to taste

Pepper to taste

2 mushrooms, chopped

1 tablespoon olive oil

Directions:

1. Preheat your air fryer to 392 degrees F.

2. Combine all ingredients in a bowl.

3. Press mixture into a small loaf pan.

4. Add pan to the air fryer basket.

5. Cook for 30 minutes.

Pork With Pears And Ginger Servings: 4

Cooking Time: 35 Minutes

Ingredients:

2 green onions, chopped

2 tablespoons avocado oil

2 pounds pork roast, sliced

½ cup coconut aminos

1 tablespoon ginger, minced

2 pears, cored and cut into wedges

¼ cup vegetable stock

1 tablespoon chives, chopped

Directions:

1. Heat up a pan with the oil over medium heat, add the onions and the meat and brown for 2 minutes on each side.

2. Add the rest of the ingredients, toss gently and bake at 390 degrees F for 30 minutes.

3. Divide the mix between plates and serve.

Nutrition Info: calories 220, fat 13.3, fiber 2, carbs 16.5, protein 8

Butter Chicken *Servings: 6*

Ingredients:

8 finely chopped garlic cloves

¼ c. chopped low-fat unsalted butter

Freshly ground black pepper

6 oz. skinless, de-boned chicken thighs

1 tsp. lemon pepper

Directions:

1. In a large slow cooker, place chicken thighs.

2. Top chicken thighs with butter evenly.

3. Sprinkle with garlic, lemon pepper and black pepper evenly.

4. Set the slow cooker on low.

5. Cover and cook for about 6 hours.

Nutrition Info: Calories: 438, Fat:28 g, Carbs:14 g, Protein:30 g, Sugars:2 g, Sodium:700 mg

Hot Chicken Wings _Servings: 4 - 5_

Ingredients:

2 tbsps. Honey

½ stick margarine

2 tbsps. Cayenne pepper

1 bottle durkee hot sauce

10 - 20 chicken wings

10 shakes Tabasco sauce

Directions:

1. In a deep pot, heat the canola oil. Deep-fry the wings until cooked, approximately 20 minutes.

2. In a medium bowl, mix the hot sauce, honey, tabasco, and cayenne pepper. Mix well.

3. Place the cooked wings on paper towels. Drain the excess oil.

4. Toss the chicken wings in the sauce until coated evenly.

Nutrition Info: Calories: 102, Fat:14 g, Carbs:55 g, Protein:23 g, Sugars:0.3 g, Sodium:340 mg

Chicken, Pasta And Snow Peas Servings: 1 - 2

Ingredients:

Fresh ground pepper

2 ½ c. penne pasta

1 standard jar tomato and basil pasta sauce 1 c. halved and trimmed snow peas

1 lb. chicken breasts

1 tsp. olive oil

Directions:

1. In a medium frying pan, heat the olive oil. Season the chicken breasts with salt and pepper. Cook the chicken breasts until cooked through for approximately 5 – 7 minutes each side.

2. Cook the pasta according to instructions on package. Cook the snow peas with the pasta.

3. Scoop 1 cup of the pasta water. Drain the pasta and peas, set aside.

4. Once the chicken is cooked, slice diagonally.

5. Add the chicken back to the frying pan. Add the pasta sauce. If the mixture seems dry.

6. Add some of the pasta water to desired consistency. Heat together.

7. Divide into bowls and serve immediately.

Nutrition Info: Calories: 140, Fat:17 g, Carbs:52 g, Protein:34 g, Sugars:2.3 g, Sodium:400 mg

378. Meatball Servings: 4

Cooking Time: 15 Minutes

Ingredients:

Cooking spray

2 lb. lean ground beef

¼ cup onion, minced

2 cloves garlic, minced

2 tablespoons parsley, chopped

Pepper to taste

½ teaspoon red pepper flakes

1 teaspoon Italian seasoning

Directions:

1. Spray your air fryer basket with oil.

2. In a bowl, mix the remaining ingredients.

3. Form meatballs from the mixture.

4. Add to the air fryer basket.

5. Cook for 15 minutes, shaking once or twice.

Apricot Chicken Wings _Servings: 3 - 4_

Ingredients:

1 medium jar apricot preserve

1 package Lipton onion dry soup mix

1 medium bottle Russian dressing

2 lbs. chicken wings

Directions:

1. Pre-heat the oven to 350°F.

2. Rinse and pat dry the chicken wings.

3. Place the chicken wings on a baking pan, single layer.

4. Bake for 45 – 60 minutes, turning halfway.

5. In a medium bowl, combine the Lipton soup mix, apricot preserve and Russian dressing.

6. Once the wings are cooked, toss with the sauce, until the pieces are coated.

7. Serve immediately with a side dish.

Nutrition Info: Calories: 162, Fat:17 g, Carbs:76 g, Protein:13 g, Sugars:24 g, Sodium:700 mg

Chicken Thighs <u>Servings: 4</u>

Cooking Time: 20 Minutes

Ingredients:

4 chicken thigh fillets

2 teaspoons olive oil

1 teaspoon garlic powder

1 teaspoon paprika

Pepper to taste

Directions:

1. Preheat your air fryer to 400 degrees F.

2. Coat chicken with oil.

3. Sprinkle both sides of chicken with garlic powder, paprika and pepper.

4. Air fry for 20 minutes.

Crispy Chicken Tenders *Servings: 4*

Cooking Time: 10 Minutes

Ingredients:

1 lb. chicken tenders

1 tablespoon olive oil

Breading

¼ cup breadcrumbs

1 teaspoon paprika

Pepper to taste

¼ teaspoon garlic powder

¼ teaspoon onion powder

Pinch cayenne pepper

Directions:

1. Preheat your air fryer to 390 degrees F.

2. Coat chicken with olive oil.

3. In a bowl, combine breading ingredients.

4. Cover chicken with breading.

5. Place in the air fryer basket.

6. Cook for 3 to 5 minutes.

7. Flip and cook for another 3 minutes.

Champion Chicken Pockets _Servings: 4_

Ingredients:

½ c. chopped broccoli

2 halved whole wheat pita bread rounds

¼ c. bottled reduced-fat ranch salad dressing ¼ c. chopped pecans or walnuts

1 ½ c. chopped cooked chicken

¼ c. plain low-fat yogurt

¼ c. shredded carrot

Directions:

1. In a small bowl stir together yogurt and ranch salad dressing.

2. In a medium bowl combine chicken, broccoli, carrot, and, if desired, nuts. Pour yogurt mixture over chicken; toss to coat.

3. Spoon chicken mixture into pita halves.

Nutrition Info: Calories: 384, Fat:11.4 g, Carbs:7.4 g, Protein:59.3 g, Sugars:1.3 g, Sodium:368.7 mg

Stovetop Barbecued Chicken Bites <u>Servings: 4</u>

Ingredients:

1 diced medium bell pepper

1 tbsp. canola oil

1 c. tangy, spicy, and sweet barbecue sauce Freshly ground black pepper

1 diced medium onion

1 lb. de-boned skinless chicken breasts

3 minced garlic cloves

Directions:

1. Wash chicken breasts and pat dry. Cut into bite-sized chunks.

2. Heat oil in a large sauté pan over medium heat. Add chicken, onion, garlic, and bell pepper, and cook, stirring, for 5 minutes.

3. Add the barbecue sauce and stir to combine. Reduce heat to medium-low and cover pan. Cook, stirring frequently, until chicken is fully cooked, about 15 minutes.

4. Remove from heat. Season to taste with freshly ground black pepper and serve immediately.

Nutrition Info: Calories: 191, Fat:5 g, Carbs:8 g, Protein:27 g, Sugars:0 g, Sodium:480 mg

Chicken And Radish Mix Servings: 4

Ingredients:

10 halved radishes

1 tbsp. organic olive oil

2 tbsps. Chopped chives

1 c. low-sodium chicken stock

4 chicken things

Black pepper

Directions:

1. Heat up a pan with all the oil over medium-high heat, add chicken, season with black pepper and brown for 6 minutes on either side.

2. Add stock and radishes, reduce heat to medium and simmer for twenty minutes.

3. Add the chives, toss, divide between plates and serve.

4. Enjoy!

Nutrition Info: Calories: 247, Fat:10 g, Carbs:12 g, Protein:22 g, Sugars:1.1 g, Sodium:673 mg

Chicken Katsu *Servings: 4*

Cooking Time: 20 Minutes

Ingredients:

Katsu Sauce

2 tablespoons soy sauce

½ cup ketchup

1 tablespoon sherry

1 tablespoon brown sugar

2 teaspoons Worcestershire sauce

1 teaspoon garlic, minced

Chicken

1 lb. chicken breast fillet, sliced

Pepper to taste

Pinch garlic powder

1 tablespoon olive oil

1 ½ cups breadcrumbs

Cooking spray

Directions:

1. Combine katsu sauce ingredients in a bowl. Set aside.

2. Preheat your air fryer to 350 degrees F.

3. Season chicken with pepper.

4. Coat chicken with oil and dredge with breadcrumbs.

5. Place in the air fryer basket.

6. Spray with oil.

7. Cook in the air fryer for 10 minutes per side.

8. Serve with sauce.

Chicken And Sweet Potato Stew *Servings: 4*

Cooking Time: 40 Minutes

Ingredients:

1 tablespoon extra virgin olive oil

2 garlic cloves, sliced

1 white onion, chopped

14 ounces (397 g) tomatoes, chopped

2 tablespoons chopped rosemary leaves

Sea salt and ground black pepper, to taste

4 free-range skinless chicken thighs

4 sweet potatoes, peeled and cubed

2 tablespoons basil leaves

Directions:

1. Preheat the oven to 375°F (190ºC).

2. Heat the olive oil in a nonstick skillet over medium heat until shimmering.

3. Add the garlic and onion to the skillet and sauté for 5 minutes or until fragrant and the onion is translucent.

4. Add the tomatoes, rosemary, salt, and ground black pepper and cook for 15 minutes or until lightly thickened.

5. Arrange the chicken thighs and sweet potatoes on a baking sheet, then pour the mixture in the skillet over the chicken and sweet potatoes. Stir to coat well. Pour in enough water to make sure the liquid cover the chicken and sweet potatoes.

6. Bake in the preheated oven for 20 minutes or until the internal temperature of the chicken reaches at least 165ºF (74ºC).

7. Remove the baking sheet from the oven and pour them in a large bowl. Sprinkle with basil and serve.

Nutrition Info: calories: 297 ; fat: 8.7g ; protein: 22.2g ; carbs: 33.1g ; fiber: 6.5g ; sugar: 9.3g; sodium: 532mg

Rosemary Beef Ribs *Servings: 4*

Cooking Time: 2 Hours

Ingredients:

1½ pounds (680 g) boneless beef short ribs

½ teaspoon garlic powder

1 teaspoon salt

½ teaspoon freshly ground black pepper

2 tablespoons olive oil

2 cups low-sodium beef broth

1 cup red wine

4 sprigs rosemary

Directions:

1. Preheat the oven to 350ºF (180ºC).

2. On a clean work surface, rub the short ribs with garlic powder, salt, and black pepper. Let stand for 10 minutes.

3. Heat the olive oil in an oven-safe skillet over medium-high heat.

4. Add the short ribs and sear for 5 minutes or until well browned.

Flip the ribs halfway through. Transfer the ribs onto a plate and set aside.

5. Pour the beef broth and red wine into the skillet. Stir to combine well and bring to a boil. Turn down the heat to low and simmer for 10

minutes until the mixture reduces to two thirds.

6. Put the ribs back to the skillet. Add the rosemary sprigs. Put the skillet lid on, then braise in the preheated oven for 2 hours until the internal temperature of the ribs reads 165ºF (74ºC).

7. Transfer the ribs to a large plate. Discard the rosemary sprigs.

Pour the cooking liquid over and serve warm.

Nutrition Info: calories: 731 ; fat: 69.1g ; carbs: 2.1g ; fiber: 0g ; protein: 25.1g ; sodium: 781mg

Chicken, Bell Pepper & Spinach Frittata

Servings: 8

Ingredients:

¾ c. frozen chopped spinach

¼ tsp. garlic powder

¼ c. chopped red onion

1 1/3 c. finely chopped cooked chicken

8 eggs

Freshly ground black pepper

1½ c. chopped and seeded red bell pepper

Directions:

1. Grease a large slow cooker.

2. In a bowl, add eggs, garlic powder and black pepper and beat well.

3. Place remaining ingredients into prepared slow cooker.

4. Pour egg mixture over chicken mixture and gently, stir to combine.

5. Cover and cook for about 2-3 hours.

Nutrition Info: Calories: 250.9, Fat:16.3 g, Carbs:10.8 g, Protein:16.2 g, Sugars:4 g, Sodium:486 mg

Roast Chicken Dal *Servings: 4*

Ingredients:

15 oz. rinsed lentils

¼ c. low-fat plain yogurt

1 minced small onion

4 c. de-boned, skinless and roasted chicken 2 tsps. Curry powder

1 ½ tsps. Canola oil

14 oz. fire-roasted diced tomatoes

¼ tsp. salt

Directions:

1. Heat oil in a large heavy saucepan over medium-high heat.

2. Add onion and cook, stirring, until softened but not browned, 3 to 4 minutes.

3. Add curry powder and cook, stirring, until combined with the onion and intensely aromatic, 20 to 30 seconds.

4. Stir in lentils, tomatoes, chicken and salt and cook, stirring often, until heated through.

5. Remove from the heat and stir in yogurt. Serve immediately.

Nutrition Info: Calories: 307, Fat:6 g, Carbs:30 g, Protein:35 g, Sugars:0.1 g, Sodium:361 mg

Chicken Taquitos _Servings: 6_

Cooking Time: 20 Minutes

Ingredients:

1 teaspoon vegetable oil

1 onion, chopped

2 tablespoon green chili, chopped

1 clove garlic, minced

1 cup chicken, cooked

2 tablespoons hot sauce

½ cup reduced-sodium cheese blend

Pepper to taste

Corn tortillas, warmed

Cooking spray

Directions:

1. Pour into a pan over medium heat.

2. Cook onion, green chili and garlic for 5 minutes, stirring often.

3. Stir in the rest of the ingredients except tortillas.

4. Cook for 3 minutes.

5. Add mixture on top of the tortillas.

6. Roll up the tortillas.

7. Preheat your air fryer to 400 degrees F.

8. Place in the air fryer basket.

9. Cook for 10 minutes.

10. .

Oregano Pork _Servings: 4_

Cooking Time: 8 Hours

Ingredients:

2 pounds pork roast, sliced

2 tablespoons oregano, chopped

¼ cup balsamic vinegar

1 cup tomato paste

1 tablespoon sweet paprika

1 teaspoon onion powder

2 tablespoons chili powder

2 garlic cloves, minced

A pinch of salt and black pepper

Directions:

1. In your slow cooker, combine the roast with the oregano, the vinegar and the other ingredients, toss, put the lid on and cook on Low for 8 hours.

2. Divide everything between plates and serve.

Nutrition Info: calories 300, fat 5, fiber 2, carbs 12, protein 24

Chicken And Avocado Bake Servings: 4

Ingredients:

2 thinly sliced green onion stalks

Mashed avocado

170 g non-fat Greek yogurt

1 ¼ g salt

4 chicken breasts

15 g blackened seasoning

Directions:

1. Start by putting your chicken breast in a plastic zip lock bag with the blackened seasoning. Close and shake, then marinate for about 2-5 minutes.

2. As your chicken is marinating, go ahead and put your Greek Yogurt, mashed avocado, and salt in your blender and pulse until smooth.

3. Place a large skillet or cast-iron pan on the stove at medium heat, oil the pan and cook the chicken until it is cooked through. You'll need about 5 minutes on each side. However, try not to dry the juices and plate it as soon as the meat is cooked.

4. Top with the yogurt mixture.

Nutrition Info: Calories: 296, Fat:13.5 g, Carbs:6.6 g, Protein:35.37 g, Sugars:0.8 g, Sodium:173 mg

Five-spice Roasted Duck Breasts Servings: 4

Ingredients:

1 tsp. five-spice powder

¼ tsp. cornstarch

2 orange juice and zest

1 tbsp. reduced-sodium soy sauce

2 lbs. de-boned duck breast

½ tsp. kosher salt

2 tsps. Honey

Directions:

1. Preheat oven to 375 0F.

2. Place duck skin-side down on a cutting board. Trim off all excess skin that hangs over the sides. Turnover and make three parallel, diagonal cuts in the skin of each breast, cutting through the fat but not into the meat. Sprinkle both sides with five-spice powder and salt.

3. Place the duck skin-side down in an ovenproof skillet over medium-low heat.

4. Cook until the fat is melted and the skin is golden brown, about 10 minutes. Transfer the duck to a plate; pour off all the fat from the pan. Return the duck to the pan skin-side up and transfer to the oven.

5. Roast the duck for 10 to 15 minutes for medium, depending on the size of the breast, until a thermometer inserted into the thickest part registers 150 0F.

6. Transfer to a cutting board; let rest for 5 minutes.

7. Pour off any fat remaining in the pan (take care, the handle will still be hot); place the pan over medium-high heat and add orange juice and honey. Bring to a simmer, stirring to scrape up any browned bits.

8. Add orange zest and soy sauce and continue to cook until the sauce is slightly reduced, about 1 minute. Stir cornstarch mixture then whisk into the sauce; cook, stirring, until slightly thickened, 1

minute.

9. Remove the duck skin and thinly slice the breast meat. Drizzle with the orange sauce.

Nutrition Info: Calories: 152, Fat:2 g, Carbs:8 g, Protein:24 g, Sugars:5 g, Sodium:309 mg

Pork Chops With Tomato Salsa *Servings: 4*

Cooking Time: 15 Minutes

Ingredients:

4 pork chops

1 tablespoon olive oil

4 scallions, chopped

1 teaspoon cumin, ground

½ tablespoon hot paprika

1 teaspoon garlic powder

A pinch of sea salt and black pepper

1 small red onion, chopped

2 tomatoes, cubed

2 tablespoons lime juice

1 jalapeno, chopped

¼ cup cilantro, chopped

1 tablespoon lime juice

Directions:

1. Heat up a pan with the oil over medium heat, add the scallions and sauté for 5 minutes.

2. Add the meat, cumin paprika, garlic powder, salt and pepper, toss, cook for 5 minutes on each side and divide between plates.

3. In a bowl, combine the tomatoes with the remaining ingredients, toss, divide next to the pork chops and serve.

Nutrition Info: calories 313, fat 23.7, fiber 1.7, carbs 5.9, protein 19.2

Tuscan Chicken With Tomatoes, Olives, And Zucchini

Servings: 4

Cooking Time: 20 Minutes

Ingredients:

4 boneless, skinless chicken breast halves, pounded to ½- to ¾-inch thickness

1 teaspoon garlic powder

½ teaspoon sea salt

⅛ teaspoon freshly ground black pepper

2 tablespoons extra-virgin olive oil

2 cups cherry tomatoes

½ cup sliced green olives

1 zucchini, chopped

¼ cup dry white wine

Directions:

1. On a clean work surface, rub the chicken breasts with garlic powder, salt, and ground black pepper.

2. Heat the olive oil in a nonstick skillet over medium-high heat until shimmering.

3. Add the chicken and cook for 16 minutes or until the internal temperature reaches at least 165ºF (74ºC). Flip the chicken halfway through the cooking time. Transfer to a large plate and cover with aluminum foil to keep warm.

4. Add the tomatoes, olives, and zucchini to the skillet and sauté for 4 minutes or until the vegetables are soft.

5. Add the white wine to the skillet and simmer for 1 minutes.

6. Remove the aluminum foil and top the chicken with the vegetables and their juices, then serve warm.

Nutrition Info: calories: 172 ; fat: 11.1g ; protein: 8.2g ; carbs: 7.9g ; fiber: 2.1g ; sugar: 4.2g ; sodium: 742mg

Pork Salad *Servings: 4*

Cooking Time: 10 Minutes

Ingredients:

1-pound pork stew meat, cut into strips

3 tablespoons olive oil

4 scallions, chopped

2 tablespoons lemon juice

2 tablespoons balsamic vinegar

2 cups mixed salad greens

1 avocado, peeled, pitted and roughly cubed 1 cucumber, sliced

2 tomatoes, cubed

A pinch of salt and black pepper

Directions:

1. Heat up a pan with 2 tablespoons of oil over medium heat, add the scallions, the meat and the lemon juice, toss and cook for 10 minutes.

2. In a salad bowl, combine the salad greens with the meat and the remaining ingredients, toss and serve.

Nutrition Info: calories 225, fat 6.4, fiber 4, carbs 8, protein 11

Lime Pork And Green Beans *Servings: 4*

Cooking Time: 40 Minutes

Ingredients:

2 pounds pork stew meat, cubed

2 tablespoons avocado oil

½ cup green beans, trimmed and halved

2 tablespoons lime juice

1 cup coconut milk

1 tablespoon rosemary, chopped

A pinch of salt and black pepper

Directions:

1. Heat up a pan with the oil over medium heat, add the meat and brown for 5 minutes.

2. Add the rest of the ingredients, toss gently, bring to a simmer and cook over medium heat for 35 minutes more.

3. Divide the mix between plates and serve.

Nutrition Info: calories 260, fat 5, fiber 8, carbs 9, protein 13

Chicken Breast *Servings: 4*

Cooking Time: 20 Minutes

Ingredients:

4 chicken breast fillets

½ teaspoon dried oregano

½ teaspoon garlic powder

Pepper to taste

Cooking spray

Directions:

1. Season chicken with oregano, garlic powder and pepper.

2. Spray with oil.

3. Place in the air fryer basket.

4. Air fry at 360 degrees F for 10 minutes per side.

Pork With Chili Zucchinis And Tomatoes

Servings: 4

Cooking Time: 35 Minutes

Ingredients:

2 tomatoes, cubed

2 pounds pork stew meat, cubed

4 scallions, chopped

2 tablespoons olive oil

1 zucchini, sliced

Juice of 1 lime

2 tablespoons chili powder

½ tablespoons cumin powder

A pinch of sea salt and black pepper

Directions:

1. Heat up a pan with the oil over medium heat, add the scallions and sauté for 5 minutes.

2. Add the meat and brown for 5 minutes more.

3. Add the tomatoes and the other ingredients, toss, cook over medium heat for 25 minutes more, divide between plates and serve.

Nutrition Info: calories 300, fat 5, fiber 2, carbs 12, protein 14

Pork With Olives _Servings: 4_

Cooking Time: 40 Minutes

Ingredients:

1 yellow onion, chopped

4 pork chops

2 tablespoons olive oil

1 tablespoon sweet paprika

2 tablespoons balsamic vinegar

¼ cup kalamata olives, pitted and chopped

1 tablespoon cilantro, chopped

A pinch of sea salt and black pepper

Directions:

1. Heat up a pan with the oil over medium heat, add the onion and sauté for 5 minutes.

2. Add the meat and brown for 5 minutes more.

3. Add the rest of the ingredients, toss, cook over medium heat for 30 minutes, divide between plates and serve.

Nutrition Info: calories 280, fat 11, fiber 6, carbs 10, protein 21

Dill And Salmon Pâté

Servings: 4

Cooking Time: 0 Minutes

Ingredients:

six ounces cooked salmon, bones and skin removed 1 Tablespoon chopped fresh dill

½ Teaspoon sea salt

¼ cup heavy (whipping) cream

Directions:

1. Take a blender or a food processor (or instead a large bowl using a mixer), mix the lemon zest, salmon, heavy cream, dill, and salt.

2. Blend till you attain the proper consistency for the smoothie.

Nutrition Info: Carbohydrate 0.4g Protein; 25.8g Total Fat: 12g Calories: 199 Cholesterol: 0.0mg Fiber: 0.8g Sodium: 296mg

Chai Spice Baked Apples *Servings: 5*

Cooking Time: 3 Hours

Ingredients:

5 apples

½ cup water

½ cup crushed pecans (optional)

¼ cup melted coconut oil

1 teaspoon ground cinnamon

½ teaspoon ground ginger

¼ teaspoon ground cardamom

¼ teaspoon ground cloves

Directions:

1. Core each apple, and peel off a thin strip from the top of each.

2. Add the water to the slow cooker. Gently place each apple upright along the bottom.

3. In a small bowl, stir together the pecans (if using), coconut oil, cinnamon, ginger, cardamom, and cloves.

4. Drizzle the mixture over the tops of the apples.

5. Cover the cooker and set to high. Cook for 2 to 3 hours, until the apples soften, and serve.

Nutrition Info: Calories: 217Total Fat: 12gTotal Carbs: 30gSugar: 22g Fiber: 6g Protein: 0gSodium: 0mg

Peach Crisp *Servings: 6*

Cooking Time: 20 Minutes

Ingredients:

Filling:

6 peaches, sliced in half

1 tablespoon coconut sugar

1 teaspoon ground cinnamon

½ tablespoon butter, sliced into cubes

Topping:

½ cup all purpose flour

½ cup coconut sugar

¼ teaspoon cinnamon powder

¼ cup vegan butter, sliced into cubes

Directions:

1. Add peaches to a small cake pan.

2. Stir in the rest of the filling ingredients.

3. In a bowl, mix the topping ingredients.

4. Spread topping over the peach mixture.

5. Air fry at 350 degrees F for 20 minutes.

Peach Dip Servings: 2

Cooking Time: 0 Minute

Ingredients:

½ cup nonfat: yogurt

1 cup peaches, chopped

A pinch of cinnamon powder

A pinch of nutmeg, ground

Directions:

1. In a bowl, combine the yogurt while using the peaches, cinnamon and nutmeg.

2. Whisk and divide into small bowls and serve.

Nutrition Info: Calories: 165Fat: 2gFiber: 3gCarbs: 14gProtein: 13g

Carrot And Pumpkin Seed Crackers *Servings: 40 Crackers*

Cooking Time: 15 Minutes

Ingredients:

1⅓ cups pumpkin seeds

½ cup packed shredded carrot (about 1 carrot) 3 tablespoons chopped fresh dill

¼ teaspoon sea salt

2 tablespoons extra-virgin olive oil

Directions:

1. Preheat the oven to 350ºF (180ºC). Line a baking sheet with parchment paper.

2. Ground the pumpkin seeds in a food processor, then add the carrot, dill, salt, and olive oil to the food processor and pulse to combine well.

3. Pour them in the prepared baking sheet, then shape the mixture into a rectangle with a spatula.

4. Line a sheet of parchment paper over the rectangle, then flatten the rectangle to about ⅛ inch thick with a rolling pin.

5. Remove the parchment paper lined over the rectangle, then score it into 40 small rectangles with a sharp knife.

6. Arrange the baking sheet in the preheated oven and bake for 15 minutes or until golden browned and crispy.

7. Transfer the crackers on a large plate and allow to cool for a few minutes before serving.

Nutrition Info: (4 crackers)calories: 130 ; fat: 11.9g ; protein: 5.1g ; carbs: 3.8g ; fiber: 1.0g ; sugar: 0g; sodium: 66mg

Avocado Fries _Servings: 8_

Cooking Time: 10 Minutes

Ingredients:

2 avocados, sliced into strips

Dry mixture

½ cup breadcrumbs

½ teaspoon onion powder

1 teaspoon garlic powder

½ teaspoon paprika powder

½ teaspoon turmeric powder

Wet mixture

½ cup flour

½ teaspoon paprika powder

½ teaspoon turmeric powder

½ cup almond milk

1 teaspoon hot sauce

Directions:

1. Mix dry mixture ingredients in a bowl.

2. In another bowl, combine wet mixture ingredients.

3. Dip each avocado strip into wet mixture, then cover with dry mixture.

4. Add to the air fryer basket.

5. Cook in the air fryer for 5 minutes.

6. Flip and cook for another 5 minutes.

www.ingramcontent.com/pod-product-compliance
Lightning Source LLC
Chambersburg PA
CBHW071817080526
44589CB00012B/819